Lecture Notes in Medical Informatics

Edited by O. Rienhoff and D.A.B. Lindberg

43

L. Hothorn (Ed.)

Statistical Methods in Toxicology

Proceedings of a Workshop during EUROTOX '90
Leipzig, Germany, September 12–14, 1990

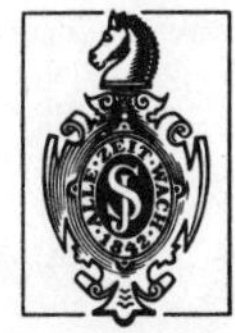

Springer-Verlag
Berlin Heidelberg New York London Paris
Tokyo Hong Kong Barcelona Budapest

Editor
Ludwig Hothorn
German Cancer Research Center Heidelberg
Institute of Epidemiology and Biometry
Im Neuenheimer Feld 280, 6900 Heidelberg, FRG

ISBN 3-540-53621-3 Springer-Verlag Berlin Heidelberg New York
ISBN 0-387-53621-3 Springer-Verlag New York Heidelberg Berlin

Printed in Germany

Printing and binding: Druckhaus Beltz, Hemsbach/Bergstr.
2127/3140-543210 – Printed on acid-free paper

Contents

Biostatistical analysis of embryo – toxicity studies

General principles in biostatistical analysis of toxicological studies

Modern Statistical Methods in Toxicology - An overview

Ludwig Hothorn
German Cancer Research Center, Department Biostatistics, P.O. B. 101949, D-6900 Heidelberg, Germany

The last discussion on statistical methods in toxicology took place during the EUROTOX '81 Dublin meeting (five papers by Weil, Peto, Gad, Tattersal and Lewi & Marsboom see Chambers, Chambers, 1981). During the past decade, a rapid development of statistical methods for toxicological studies could be observed. This development was supported by the standardization of several toxicological studies due to national (e.g., Bundeschemikaliengesetz, anonymous, 1980) or international guidelines (e.g., OECD Guidelines for testing of chemicals, anonymous, 1981 or EC Guidelines, anonymous, 1983). For this reason, during the EUROTOX '90 conference a special workshop on statistical methods in toxicology was organized. This workshop was mainly intended to provide a contribution to the demand for "appropriate statistical analysis" within the guidelines of the so-called "regulatory toxicology".
For this reason four topics were discussed:

Topic 1: Biostatistical analysis of mutagenicity assays

In an invited paper, Schumacher and Schmoor (Freiburg i. Br., Germany) gave an overview on experimental design and statistical evaluation of the commonly used Ames assay. The essential problem of the interaction of a monotonic mutagenic effect with a possible high-dose toxicity effect within the Ames assay was discussed in detail based on three related approaches.
Leimer, Peil and Ellenberger (Ingelheim, Germany) discussed the biostatistical analysis of the micronucleus assay using the Fisher-Pitman permutation test. This particular method of analysis was advocated due to the small number of micronucleus counts, frequent number of tied values and an unknown distribution.
In two papers, Lehn and Rettig (Darmstadt, Germany) illustrated the modelling of the time-dependent structure of the HGPRT assay based on a Markov chain model. Using this model, they proposed a test for mutagenicity, and presented simulation results describing the size and power of this test.
In a poster, Piegorsch and Zeiger (Research Triangle Park, U.S.A.) described an inference method for measuring intra-assay agreement based on a Kappa coefficient. Using

Ames assay data on 239 chemicals from the U.S. National Toxicology Program, the authors could show a significant positive intra-assay agreement, both as a whole and for pertinent subdivisions of the data.
As an addenum an overview paper by Vollmar and Edler (Mannheim & Heidelberg, Germany) on several approaches for the biostatistical analysis of the Ames assay was included in this chapter.
Within this topic, several new ideas for the biostatistical evaluation of mutagenicity test data were discussed. More traditional approaches are given in a book by (Kirkland, 1989) based on the mainly use of variance analysis after endpoint transformation.

Topic 2: Biostatistical analysis of Long-term carcinogenicity studies

In an invited paper, Kaufmann (Berlin, Germany) gave an overview on the practical analysis of mortality and tumour data within long-term carcinogenicity studies based on parametric test statistics. With real-data examples the effect of subdivisions of tumour data related to time sections or tumour sites in detail was discussed.
Ehrenberg (Stockholm, Sweden) discussed several types of mathematical models concerning initiating and promoting effects of carcinogens. The problem of model validity and low-dose extrapolation was described based on several real-data examples. It was pointed out that the accuracy is limited on the usual experimental design which uses only three or four dose groups. The problems in estimation a thereshold in dose-response relationships for mutation and cancer was discussed based on real data examples by Granath (Stockholm, Sweden).

An overview of biostatistical methods for the evaluation of long-term carcinogenicity studies present within the book of Gart et.al. (1986) and Vollmar (1986).

Topic 3: Biostatistical analysis of embryo-toxicity studies

In an invited paper, Piegorsch (Research Triangle Park, U.S.A.) reviewed several approaches for the analysis of binomial endpoints in embryo-toxicity studies, e.g. number of malformed fetuses/number of all fetuses. It was stressed that the litter should be regarded as the appropriate experimental unit for quantitative analysis in studies for teratogenic or heritable mutagenic effects. Approaches for per-litter analysis involving extra–binomial proportion responses range from non–parametric analyses over resampling methods to models involving generalized binomial distributions. Rosenkranz (Frankfurt, Germany) discussed the problem of per–litter analysis for continous data, e.g. fetus weights. In comparison with the variance analysis approach according to (Healy, 1972) several maximum likelihood approaches were proposed.

Meister (Berlin, Germany) discussed another source of variability related to strain–differences. It was demonstrated how a biostatistical model for onset and speed of embryonic development (number of somites) can be assessed and differences in the analyzed growth process can be used to explain the observed strain–differences. Furthermore a comparison of the within and between litter variation in time was shown. More traditional approaches to the biostatistical analysis of embryo–toxicity studies are given by Gaylor (1978) or Gad and Weil (1986).

Topic 4: General principles in biostatistical analysis of toxicological studies

In an invited paper, Hothorn (Heidelberg, Germany) discussed the multiplicity problem occuring in testing in toxicology. He gave an overview on the typical one–way design "control versus k treatment or dose groups". For this kind of hypotheses formulation, biostatistical methods should be used that guarantee a minimum type II error and that control the type I error for each experiment. In this sense two–sample versus k–sample testing, tests (single decision problem), versus procedures (multiple decision problem), simultaneous versus sequentially rejective procedures were compared. The behaviour in data situation for the typically used Dunnett, (1955) procedure was described such as the violation of the normal distribution, variance heterogeneity assumption. For different types of endpoints appropriate comparison procedures with and without the assumption of a monotonic dose–response relationship were discussed. On the other hand, a paper of Maul (Nancy, France) was directed to the application of the so–called generalized linear models to dichotomous, count or continous data for parameter estimation and effect testing in toxicological dose–response relationships. Model fitting and evaluation was illustrated by some data examples. Repeto (Verona, Italy) described the application of mixed model analysis of variance for the design TREATMENT TIME in behavioural toxicity studies.
Unkelbach (Darmstadt & Wiesbaden, Germany) discussed the need of software validation in regulatory toxicology. In the consequence of the GLP principles, all software used for a toxicological study is subject to a quality assurance programme of the

laboratories. Difficulties with the validation of numerical and statistical algorithms were discussed in detail.

Textbooks on general statistical methods in toxicology are available; e.g., Salsbury, (1984) and Horn and Hothorn, (1990).

References

anonymous (1980) Gesetz zum Schutz vor gefährlichen Stoffen. (Bundeschemikaliengesetz, Bundesdrucksache Nr. 376/80).

anonymous (1981) OECD guidelines for testing of chemicals. OECD, Paris.

anonymous (1983) Empfehlungen des Rates vom 26.10.1983 zu den Versuchen mit Arzneimitteln (EWG 831517). In: Pharm. Ind. 45: 1248–1261.

Chambers PL and Chambers CM (ed.) (1981) New Toxicology for Old: Statistics in Toxicology. Archives of Toxicology Suppl. 5, pp. 237–271.

Gad S and Weil CS (1986) Statistics and Experimental Design for Toxicologists. Telford Press, Caldwell, NJ.

Gaylor DM (1978) Methods and concepts of biometrics applied to teratology. In: Handbook of Teratology (ed.: Wilson, J.G.) Vol. 4, Plenum Press, New York.

Healy MRJ (1972) Animal litters as experimental units. Appl. Statistics 21: 155–159.

Horn M and Hothorn L (1990) Grundlagen der Statistik für Toxikologen. Verlag Gesundheit 2nd ed. 1–245.

Gart JJ et al. (1986) The design and analysis of long-term animal experiments. IARC Sci Publ No 79 IARC Lyon, 1–219.

Kirkland DJ (ed.) (1989) Statistical evaluation of mutagenicity test data. Cambridge University Press. Cambridge, 1–292.

Salsbury DS (1986) Statistics for toxicologists. Marcel Dekker, Inc. New York.

Vollmar J (ed.) (1986) Auswertungs- und Darstellungsmethoden. Risikoextrapolation zur Kanzerogenität. Biometrie i.d. chem.-pharm. Industrie. Vol. 3, Fischer Verlag Stuttgart, 1–183.

STATISTICAL ANALYSIS OF THE AMES ASSAY

Martin Schumacher and Claudia Schmoor
Institut für Med. Biometrie und Med. Informatik der Universität Freiburg
Stefan-Meier-Str. 26, D-7800 Freiburg

1 Introduction

The Ames or Salmonella/microsome assay (Ames et al., 1973, 1975) is the most prominent example of a short-term mutagenicity test. Originally developed and widely used for the selection of potentially mutagenic (and carcinogenic) compounds in a relatively - compared to long-term animal experiments - short period of time, it has also been used for the biological monitoring of humans exposed to environmental pollutants (Berlin et al., 1984; Margolin, 1988).

The test system of the Ames assay is based on the detection of reverse mutation from histidine requirement to histidine non-requirement as a response to mutagenic agents in specially constructed cell strains of Salmonella typhimurium. Only the so-called revertants will continue to divide and will form visible, discrete colonies. The endpoint for the evaluation is the number of revertant colonies counted on replicated plates in a dose-response experiment. Such an experiment is typically carried out with five to seven dose levels and three to five replicates for each dose level.

The two major problems associated with the Ames assay are the statistical variability and the so-called 'Muta-Tox Problem'. The first of these problems refers to the high variability of the data obtained from an Ames assay - in statistical terms refered to as 'Overdispersion' - which might among other reasons be due to the use of different strains, variations in the environment of the assay and unspecific laboratory effects. The second problem refers to the dilemma that the mutagenic effect of a compound can often be observed only at high concentrations or dose levels of that compound. On the other hand, many compounds exhibit serious toxic effects at higher dose levels interfering with the mutagenic effect. These two problems, formulated and discussed here in terms of the Ames assay, are in principle also the major problems of other short-term mutagenicity tests. Thus the considerations below on the statistical analysis of the Ames assay can also serve, at least as a rough guideline, for the statistical evaluation of mutagenicity test data in general. For comprehensive overviews we refer to Breslow and Kaldor (1986), Kirkland (1989) and Edler (1990).

In this paper, some of the statistical procedures proposed are presented. The methods are illustrated by an example and some recommendations are given.

2 Statistical model

The experimental situation of an Ames assay can be summarized as follows:

$x_1, x_2, \ldots, x_I$ denote the dose levels of the test compound in ascending order where $x_1 = 0$ serves as a control;

$n_1, n_2, \ldots, n_I$ denote the number of replicate plates at the respective dose levels and

y_{ij} denotes the observed number of revertants at the dose level x_i counted on plate j ($i = 1, \ldots, I$; $j = 1, \ldots, n_i$) which is the endpoint for the statistical evaluation of the Ames assay.

The data of a typical Ames assay are shown in table 1. The experiment comprises six dose levels (including the control) of the compound Acid Red 114 with three replicate plates for each dose level; Salmonella thyphimurium TA 98 with hamster liver activation has been used. The data are also graphically displayed in figure 1.

Table 1 Revertant colonies for Acid Red 114 (TA 98, Hamster liver activation); Source: Simpson and Margolin (1986)

Dose (µg/l)					
0	100	333	1000	3333	10000
23	27	28	41	28	16
22	23	37	37	21	19
14	21	35	43	30	13

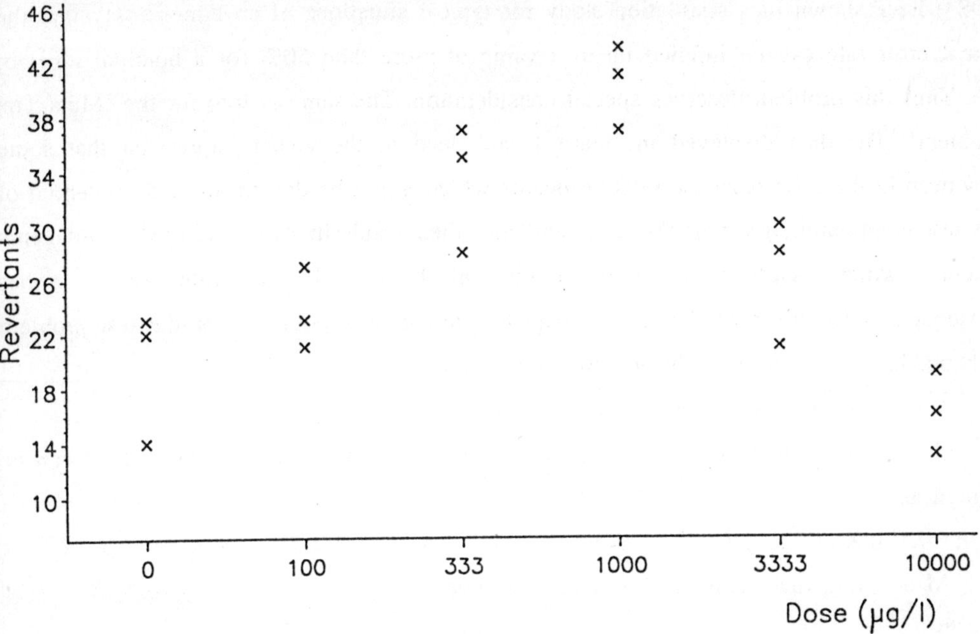

Figure 1 Revertant colonies for Acid Red 114 (TA 98, Hamster liver activation); Source: Simpson and Margolin (1986)

The statistical model is derived from the observation that the average number of microbes originally given on each plate, say N_0, is usually in the order of magnitude of 10^6 to 10^8, whereas the probability of a backmutation and the generation of a visible colony for each microbe exposed to dose level x_i, denoted by $P(x_i)$, is usually very small (approximately 10^{-9} to 10^{-5}). Thus a natural starting point would be the assumption of a Poisson distribution for the observed counts, represented by the expected number of revertant counts, $\lambda_i = N_0 * P(x_i)$ at dose level x_i $(i = 1, ..., I)$.

These expected numbers of revertants can also be used for the formulation of the test problem of interest: The null-hypothesis H_0 of no mutagenic effect of the test compound can be expressed as

$$H_0 : \lambda_1 = \lambda_2 = ... = \lambda_I$$

The impact of the two major problems already mentioned in the introduction section on the statistical analysis can be seen immediately. Overdispersion can inflate the type I error rate considerably when falsely assuming a Poisson distribution for the observed counts with the consequence that the variance should be equal to the expected values. Lin and Sanford

(1983) have shown in a simulation study for typical situations of an Ames assay that the type I error rate can be inflated up to a value of more than 50% for a nominal level of 5%. Thus this problem deserves special consideration. The same is true for the 'Muta-Tox Problem'. The data displayed in figure 1 may lead to the visual impression that some downturn in the dose-response relation occurs which might be due to the toxic potential of the test compound. Ignoring this problem may then result in overlooking the mutagenic potential which clearly leads to an inflation of the type II error rate. This also has consequences for the formulation of adequate alternative hypotheses for the test problem at hand. Instead of the straightforward formulation

$$H_1: \ \lambda_1 \leq \lambda_2 \leq \ldots \leq \lambda_I \quad \text{and} \quad \lambda_1 < \lambda_I$$

it might be more adequate to allow for a downturn, i.e., the alternative hypothesis can be written as

$$H_1: \ \lambda_1 \leq \lambda_2 \leq \ldots \leq \lambda_M \geq \ldots \geq \lambda_I \quad \text{and} \quad \lambda_1 < \lambda_M,$$

with M denoting the maximal non-toxic dose level.

3 Approaches to the statistical analyis

The statistical methods proposed for the evaluation of the Ames assay can be classified according to the way they focus attention on the problem of overdispersion and the 'Muta-Tox Problem'. A natural way would be a distinction between parametric - probably with consideration of possible overdispersion - and nonparametric methods. Much more relevant, however, is to distinguish between the ways the 'Muta-Tox Problem' is adressed. With respect to this problem, the statistical methods can be classified into three categories which are illustrated in figure 2. Category I contains those methods in which the possible toxicity is ignored or, in a more optimistic fashion, where it is assumed that toxicity does not play an important role in a particular Ames assay. Within this category, several parametric and nonparametric trend tests have been proposed which are also used in other applications. The procedures of the second category try to model the competing risks, mutagenicity and toxicity, by considering the specific biological background. These are primarily parametric procedures in which an appropriate functional form of the dose-response relationship is assumed including an additional parameter representing the toxic effect. An alternative approach which leads to the third category of statistical procedures is to consider toxicity only as a disturbing effect which superimposes the interesting mutagenic effect. In these so-called 'adaptive' or 'recursive' procedures, all data at dose levels which mainly show toxic effects are eliminated. The statistical evaluation of the mutagenic effect is then solely based on the remaining dose groups.

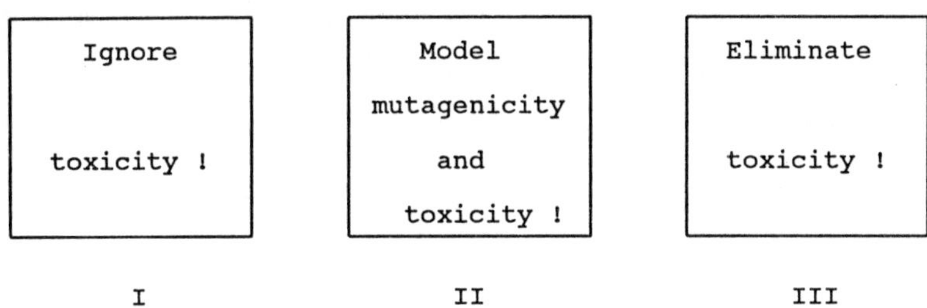

Figure 2 Classification of statistical methods with respect to the 'Muta-Tox Problem'

In the sequel, we will present some selected examples of statistical methods from each category showing the typical features and problems of these methods. This presentation is by no means intended as a comprehensive overview covering almost all statistical methods proposed so far. For such an overview we refer to the recently updated comprehensive list in this volume compiled by Vollmar and Edler (1990) which is also contained in the review paper by Edler (1990).

3.1 Statistical methods of category I

As already mentioned above, category I contains those methods where the possible toxicity is not considered to be a major problem. Snee & Irr (1981) recommended the use of simple linear regression analysis for the routine evaluation of the Ames assay. In this setting, they assumed that the expected number of revertants can be written as

$$\lambda_i = \beta_0 + \beta_1 x_i \qquad (i = 1, \ldots, I)$$

where the intercept β_0 represents the rate of spontaneous revertants and β_1 represents the interesting mutagenic potential. Clearly, such an analysis is based on the assumptions

- Normal distribution of observed counts,
- Homogeneity of variances,
- Linearity of the dose-response relationship.

Therefore, these authors recommended the use of the Box-Cox transformation $(y_{ij} + 1)^{0.15}$ for the observed counts (Box & Cox, 1964).

The test statistic for testing the null hypothesis of no mutagenic effect is based on a comparison of the estimated regression coefficient $\hat{\beta}_1$ with its standard error. In our example this leads to a test statistic of 0.46 which is associated with a p-value of 0.33. Thus, the use of the simple linear regression method yields no indication for a mutagenic effect of the compound Acid Red 114 in this assay. The estimated regression line is displayed in figure 3 underlining the poor fit of the linear regression model for these data.

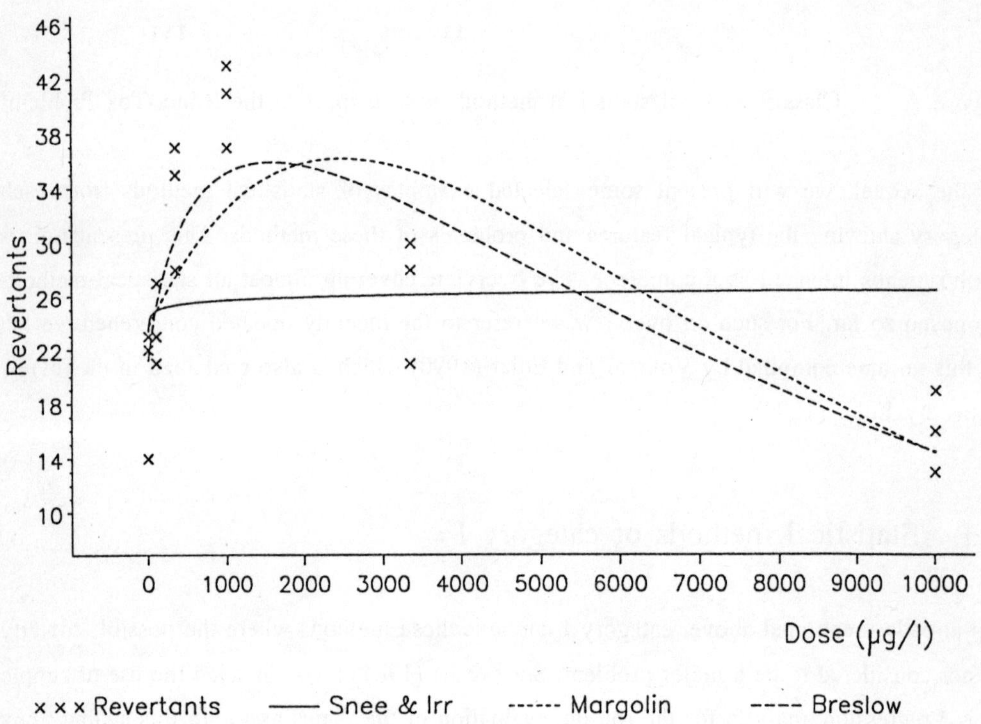

Figure 3 Fitted regression curves by applying the procedures proposed by Snee & Irr (1981), Margolin et al. (1981) and Breslow (1984)

A nonparametric method which belongs to category I is a modification of the well-known Page test (Page, 1963) which has been proposed by Wahrendorf et al. (1985) for the evaluation of the Ames assay. It is based on an overall ranking of the observed counts at all dose levels and a comparison of the groups comprising all observations at dose levels 1 to i and dose levels i+1 to I, respectively. The test statistic is the sum of the resulting I-1 Wilcoxon statistics. Wahrendorf et al. provide tables of critical values for this test statistic and formulae for a proper standardization when using an asymptotic approximation for the distribution of the test statistic. In our example, the use of the modified Page test leads to a p-value of $p = 0.6$ again indicating no mutagenic potential of the test compound. Thus, although this nonparametric approach does not have the serious drawbacks of the simple linear regression approach in the experimental situation considered, its use is clearly limited to those situations where toxicity is not a serious problem in an assay.

3.2 Statistical methods of category II

The most elaborate method specifically designed for the statistical analysis of the Ames assay has been proposed by Margolin et al. (1981). It makes use of a single-hit model for the initiation of the mutagenic effect and on the consideration of a stochastic model for the development of the microbes based on the theory of branching processes. Additionally assuming that mutagenicity and toxicity act independently of each other, these authors were led to assume the model

$$\lambda_i = (\beta_0 + \beta_1 x_i) \exp(-\gamma x_i) \qquad (i = 1, ..., I)$$

for the expected number of revertants. Again, the coefficients β_0 and β_1 represent the rate of spontaneous revertants and the mutagenic effect, respectively, whereas γ represents the toxic effect of the compound. To account for possible overdispersion Margolin et al. (1981) assumed a Negative Binominal distribution for the observed counts which implies that the variance of the observed counts at the ith dose level is equal to $\lambda_i(1 + c\lambda_i)$ where $c \geq 0$ is an additional coefficient representing the degree of overdispersion.

Simultaneous estimation of all four unknown coefficients is via the maximum likelihood method; the test statistic for testing the hypothesis of no mutagenic effect is again based on a comparison of the estimated coefficient $\hat{\beta}_1$ with its standard error. The estimated regression curve from the data in our example is displayed in figure 3. In contrast to the simple linear regression approach this curve exhibits a satisfactory fit to the observed counts; the test statistic yields a value of 3.05 associated with a p-value of $p = 0.001$ which clearly shows the mutagenic potential of the test compound under consideration. The only problem with this otherwise nice and well-founded method is that the simultaneous maximum likelihood estimation of all four parameters causes serious difficulties and is often very unstable (see also Margolin et al., 1989). Thus this method cannot be recommended for the routine evaluation of Ames test data. To circumvent this problem, Breslow (1984) proposed in a more general framework, a pragmatic approach based on the quasi-likelihood principle (McCullagh & Nelder, 1983). Instead of fully specifying the type of distribution for the observed numbers of revertants only the expected numbers are specified as

$$\log \lambda_i = \beta_0 + \beta_1 \log (x_i + 1) - \gamma x_i \qquad (i = 1, ..., I)$$

and in addition, the variance of the observed counts is assumed to have the same form as the negative binominal variance, i.e. $\lambda_i (1 + c\lambda_i)$.

The dose response function is a little bit different from the one originally proposed by Margolin et al. (1981), but this difference is negligable in practice. The coefficients have the same meaning as in the Margolin model; the estimation procedure, however, involves an extra iterative procedure for estimating c, the degree of overdispersion. This quasi-likelihood approach turned out to be very stable. Moreover, it could be shown by Moore (1986) that the estimated coefficients have the same statistical properties as usual maximum likelihood estimators.

The fitted regression curve for the data of our example is again displayed in figure 3 allowing a direct comparison with the Margolin and the linear regression approach. The test statistic yields a value of 4.67 associated with a p-value of $p = 0.0002$, which indicates an even more pronounced mutagenic effect of the test compound.

3.3 Statistical methods of category III

The basic idea in the construction of adaptive procedures is that the dose-response-function of a mutagenic chemical increases monotonically until the mutagenic effect of the test agent is dominated by toxic effects, so that the curve decreases. Therefore, it is the first step to determine that dose level up to which the curve is increasing. Then all higher dose groups are eliminated and, for the analysis of mutagenicity, a trend test based on the remaining dose levels is performed.

A reasonable approach to the determination of the maximal non-toxic dose level, say x_M, is to investigate the dose levels for toxicity successively. That is to say, the toxicity of the kth dose is examined by an appropriate statistical test. If the hypothesis of no toxicity of the kth dose is rejected by means of this test, it is concluded to eliminate the kth and all higher dose groups and to perform a trend test for mutagenicity solely on the first k-1 dose groups. Otherwise, toxicity of the $(k+1)^{th}$ dose is examined, and so on.

The critical point in this procedure is the choice of an appropriate 'toxicity test'. On one hand, one is interested in the detection of seriously toxic doses; on the other hand, no dose groups should be rejected in which the response deviates only slightly from the monotonic trend but is still higher than some responses on lower dose levels, since this would result in a loss of power of the test for mutagenicity. Special problems arise, since in the analysis of a concrete experiment it is usually not known whether the chemical was tested up to a toxic region. The choice of the significance level of the toxicity test plays an important role, particularly since this affects reduction of the significance level for the mutagenicity test necessary to control the overall size of the whole test procedure.

An adaptive parametric procedure was proposed by Bernstein et al. (1982). Here, following the suggestion of Margolin et al. (1981), the distribution of the number of revertant colonies y_{ij} is assumed to be Negative Binomial with mean λ_i and variance $\lambda_i(1 + c\lambda_i)$. Within each dose level the mean is modelled as

$\lambda_i = \beta_0 + \beta_1 x_i$,

where β_0 is the expected number of spontaneous revertants and β_1 is the slope of the dose-response-function which represents the mutagenic effect.

The assessment of possible toxic effects is based on likelihood-ratio-tests. However, as already mentioned in section 3.2, the proposed fitting algorithm using full maximum-likelihood estimation is not well-suited for routine applications. For that reason, we suggest to replace that by the quasi-likelihood approach of Breslow (1984) outlined in section 3.2. The question whether the kth dose level is toxic is then investigated in the following way: We fit the model $\lambda_i = \beta_0 + \beta_1 x_i$ to the data of the first k-1 dose levels. The estimated coefficients obtained are denoted by $\hat{\beta}_{0,\,k-1}$ and $\hat{\beta}_{1,\,k-1}$. Based on these estimates, the expected number of revertant colonies in the kth dose group is predicted by

$\tilde{y}_k = \hat{\beta}_{0,\,k-1} + \hat{\beta}_{1,\,k-1} x_k$.

This predicted number $\tilde{y}_k$ is compared to the average number of revertant colonies observed, $\bar{y}_{k.}$, in the kth dose group by using the test-statistic $\tilde{y}_k - \bar{y}_{k.}$ which follows, under the hypothesis of no toxicity of the kth dose, approximately a standard Normal distribution. If the hypothesis of no toxicity of the kth dose is rejected based on this one-sided test, the analysis of mutagenicity is performed on the basis of the first k-1 dose levels. Otherwise, the toxicity of the $(k+1)^{th}$ dose is examined, and so on.

In contrast to Bernstein et al. (1982), who proposed to start the examination of the toxic effect at the highest dose level, we have decided to investigate the toxicity of the dose levels in ascending order, starting with the 4th dose. With the former proposal one would not be able to detect the toxicity of the highest dose, if already lower dose levels show strong toxic effects. This has been confirmed by means of a Monte Carlo study where the procedure starting the examination of toxicity at the highest dose level showed lower power in nearly all situations considered.

To control the overall size of the test procedure, the correlations among the test statistics have to be taken into account. Since the parameters are fitted iteratively by the quasi likelihood procedure, the variances and covariances of the estimates cannot be specified in closed form. In order to estimate the magnitude of the correlations, we have calculated the variances and covariances in the case of ordinary least-square-estimation of the coefficients. By means of a simulation study it could be shown that the correlations, as well as the actual size of the whole test procedure, are very well approximated using the calculation in the case of ordinary least-squares-estimation of the coefficients. From this the correction of the significance level of the single mutagenicity test necessary to control the overall size of the whole test procedure can be derived. This correction strongly depends on the choice of the significance level, say α_T, of the toxixity test. The significance level of the mutagenicity test, say α_M, has to be corrected most, if the significance level of the toxicity test is chosen equal to the demanded level of the whole test procedure, say 0.05. This is due to strong correlations among the test statistics of the mutagenicity and the toxicity tests. Therefore, in order to reduce α_M as little as possible, a very low or a very high value of α_T should be used.

In the originally proposed procedure (Bernstein et al., 1982), it was suggested to choose $\alpha_T = 0.25$. That means that toxic dose levels are detected in any case, but also those dose levels will be judged as toxic, which deviate only slightly from a monotonic trend. By choosing $\alpha_T = 0.01$, only seriously toxic dose levels are eliminated. Experiments without toxicity are analyzed on the basis of all dose levels, and therefore no loss of power of the mutagenicity tests should be expected. Moreover, in our investigations it turned out that the very low level of $\alpha_T = 0.01$ is adequate to detect strong toxicity. Therefore, we have decided to choose $\alpha_T = 0.01$. More details can be found in Schmoor and Schumacher (1989).

Applying this procedure to our example, the model is first of all fitted to the data of the first 3 dose levels. To examine the toxicity of the 4th dose, the predicted value $\tilde{y}_4 = 31.92$ is compared to the average number of revertant colonies observed, $\bar{y}_{4.} = 40.3$, in the 4th dose group. This results in a value of the standardized test statistic of -2.33 associated with a p-value of $p = 0.99$, so that the 4th dose group is not eliminated. Then the model is fitted to the data of the first 4 dose groups. The inspection of the toxic effect of the 5th dose results in $\tilde{y}_5 = 38.62$ and $\bar{y}_{5.} = 26.3$. The value of the standardized toxicity test statistic is 3.03 and the corresponding p-value $p = 0.0065$, which indicates a toxic effect of the 5th dose. Therefore, the analysis of the mutagenic effect is based on the first 4 dose groups alone. This yields a p-value, adjusted for the rejection process, of $p < 0.001$. The procedure is graphically displayed in figure 4.

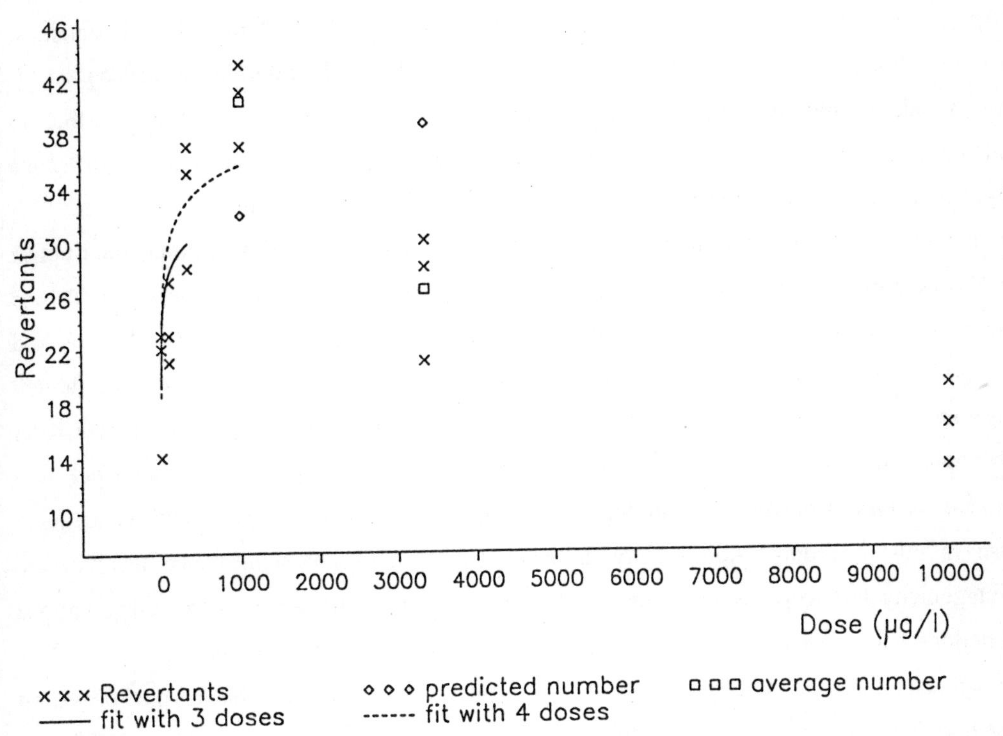

Figure 4 Graphic presentation of the parametric adaptive procedure

By constructing an analogous nonparametric procedure, the problem arises that on the basis of nonparametric procedures trend estimation and, therewith, extrapolation of trend is not feasible. Simpson and Margolin (1986) proposed a nonparametric adaptive procedure where the toxicity of the kth dose level is examined by a two-sample test, i.e., the Mann-Whitney test, where the observations of the kth dose group form one sample, and the other sample is composed of the observations of the lower dose groups. In contrast to the parametric toxicity test described above, this test does not take into account a possible existing trend within the first k-1 dose levels, because they are combined into one sample. Therefore, the nonparametric toxicity test will have far lower power than the corresponding parametric test. As a trend test for mutagenicity, the Jonckheere test (Jonckheere, 1954) is proposed. This test - applied to the first M non-toxic dose levels - is based on pairwise comparisons between dose level i and i+1 to M, for i = 1, ..., M-1, using the Mann-Whitney statistic. The resulting trend test statistic is the sum of these M(M-1)/2 Mann-Whitney statistics. Another choice would be the Page-type test proposed by Wahrendorf et al. (1985).

Again, taking into account the correlations among the test statistics, it is possible to calculate the size of the whole test procedure as well as the correction of the significance level of the mutagenicity test necessary to control the overall significance level.

In contrast to the parametric procedure, the significance level of the mutagenicity test has to be reduced the more as the significance level of the toxicity tests increases. This is due to another correlation structure among the test statistics in this procedure. Simpson and Margolin (1986) proposed a significance level of the toxicity test of $\alpha_T = 0.5$. Even though the non-parametric test is much less powerful than the parametric test, by using $\alpha_T = 0.5$ also randomly varying data are eliminated from the analysis. Since the consequence is a substantial loss of power of the mutagenicity test, we recommend a lower significance level also in this procedure. Additionally, a lower reduction of the significance level of the mutagenicity test, α_M, is necessary in this case. Monte Carlo results comprising various situations have shown that a choice of $\alpha_T = 0.1$ is a good compromise.

In our example, the toxicity test for the 4th dose level yields a p-value of p = 0.992, so the toxicity of the 5th dose is investigated. This test results in a p-value of p = 0.332, and therefore, by performing the toxicity test at significance level $\alpha_T = 0.1$, the 5th dose level remains in the model and the test is performed for the 6th dose. This leads to a p-value of p = 0.007, so the 6th dose group is eliminated and the mutagenicity test is based on the first 5 dose levels. The resulting p-value, adjusted for the rejection process, is p = 0.016.

4 Conclusions

In this paper we have presented some selected examples of statistical methods which have been proposed for the statistical analysis of the Ames assay. This presentation - although by no means intended to be comprehensive - shows the typical features of the statistical methods concerning the way the two major problems of mutagenicity data are adressed. The consideration of these typical features has led us to classify the statistical methods into the three categories I, II and III as shown in figure 2.

The limitations of statistical methods of category I are obvious. Thus their use could only be recommended for the statistical analysis of Ames assays where a priori the problem of toxicity can be ruled out. In such a case nonparametric methods such as the Page-type test (Wahrendorf et al., 1985) should be preferred. It should be mentioned that the only monograph on the statistical analysis of mutagenicity data available (Kirkland et al., 1989) solely comprises methods of category I in the corresponding chapter on the Ames and related assays (Mahon et al., 1989).

The most elaborate method also reflecting the biological background (Margolin et al., 1981) suffers from the fact that it is often very unstable and therefore cannot be recommended for routine use. The pragmatic alternative proposed by Breslow (1984) based on the quasi-likelihood principle provides a suitable alternative which also showed a good performance in a wide range of situations considered. However, it has to be recognized that - as in all other methods of category II - the toxic effect of the test compound has to be modelled and, as a consequence, that a misspecification in this modelling might compromise the statistical analysis of the mutagenic effect. The 'adaptive' procedures of category III avoid the problem of modelling the interfering toxic effect. Although a definitive assessment of the various proposals is still missing - for partial assessments cf. Schmoor and Schumacher (1989) and Simpson and Margolin (1990) - they provide an intuitively appealing and valid methodology for the statistical analysis of the Ames assay and other short-term mutagenicity tests.

5 References

Ames BN, Durston WE, Yamasaki E and Lee FD (1973) Carcinogens are mutagens: A simple test system combining liver homogenates for activation and bacteria for detection. Proceedings of the National Academy of Sciences USA 70:2281-2285

Ames BN, McCann J and Yamasaki E (1975) Methods for detecting carcinogens and mutagens with the Salmonella/mammalian microsome test. Mutation Research 31:347-364

Berlin A, Draper M, Hemminki K and Vainio H (eds) (1984) Monitoring human exposure to carcinogenic and mutagenic agents. IARC Scientific Publications No. 59 IARC Lyon

Bernstein L, Kaldor J, McCann J and Pike MC (1982) An empirical approach to the statistical analysis of mutagenesis data from the Salmonella test. Mutation Research 97:267-281

Box GEP and Cox DR (1964) An analysis of transformation. Journal of the Royal Statistic Society, Series B 26:211-252

Breslow NE (1984) Extra-Poisson variation in log-linear models. Applied Statistics 33:38-44

Breslow N and Kaldor J (1986) Statistical analysis of data from in-vitro assays of mutagenesis. IARC Scientific publications No. 83 IARC Lyon, 457-481

Edler L (1990) Biostatistical issues in short-term tests for genetic toxicology. Technical Report

Jonckheere AR (1954) A distribution-free k-sample test against ordered alternatives. Biometrika 41: 133-145

Kirkland DJ (ed) (1989) Statistical evaluation of mutagenicity test data. UKEMS subcommittee on guidelines for mutagenicity testing. Report, part III. Cambridge University Press Cambridge

Lin LIK and Sanford RL (1983) The robustness of the likelihood ratio test, the nonparametric sum rank test, and F-ratio tests when the populations are from the negative binomial familiy. Commun. Statist.-Simula. Computa. 12:523-539

Mahon G, Green M, Middleton B, Mitchell I, Robinson D and Tweats D (1989) Analysis of data from microbial colony assays. In: Kirkland DJ (ed) s.a., 26-65

Margolin BH, Kaplan N and Zeiger E (1981) Statistical analysis of the Ames Salmonella/microsome test. Proceedings of the National Academy of Sciences USA 78:3779-3783

Margolin BH, Kim BS and Risko KJ (1989) The Ames Salmonella/microsome mutagenicity assay: Issues of inference and validations. Journal of the American Statistical Association 84:651-661

Margolin BH (1988) Statistical aspects of using biological markers. Statistical Science 3:351-357

McCullagh P and Nelder JA (1983) Generalized linear models. Chapman and Hall London

Moore DF (1986) Asymptotic properties of moment estimators for overdispersed counts and proportions. Biometrika 73:583-588

Page EB (1963) Ordered hypothesis for multiple treatments: A significance test for linear ranks. Journal of the American Statistical Association 58:216-230

Schmoor C and Schumacher M (1989) Adaptive statistical procedures for the analysis of mutagenicity data. Preprint University of Freiburg

Simpson DG and Margolin BH (1986) Recursive nonparametric testing for dose-response-relationships subject to downturns at high doses. Biometrika 73:589-596

Simpson DG and Margolin BH (1990) Nonparametric testing for dose-response curves subject to downturns: Asymptotic power considerations. The Annals of Statistics 18: 373-390

Snee RD and Irr JD (1981) Design of a statistical method for the analysis of mutagenesis at the Hypoxanthine-Guanine Phosphoribozyl Transferase of cultured chinese hamster ovary cells. Mutation Research 85:77-93

Vollmar J and Edler L (1990) Tabular overview of statistical methods proposed for the analysis of Ames Salmonella Assay data. In: Lecture Notes in Medical Informatics Vol. 41 (this volume),

Wahrendorf J, Mahon GAT and Schumacher M (1985) A nonparametric approach to the statistical analysis of mutagenicity data. Mutation Research 147:5-13

STATISTICAL ANALYSIS OF THE MICRONUCLEUS TEST WITH THE FISHER-PITMAN PERMUTATION TEST

I. Leimer, H. Peil and J. Ellenberger
Division of Research and Development,
Boehringer Ingelheim KG, 6507 Ingelheim, FRG

Introduction

The micronucleus test is an in vivo genotoxicity assay for screening chemicals for chromosome-breaking effects (Schmid, 1975). The basic measurement for analysis is the number of micronucleated cells per animal in a predefined number of polychromatic erythrocytes. An increase in the frequency of micronucleated polychromatic erythrocytes relative to the controls indicates chromosomal damage induced by the substance under test.

No standard procedure for the statistical analysis of the micronucleus test has yet been established (Kirkland, 1989; MacGregor et al., 1987; PSI, 1986). Most methods depend on distributional assumptions, which are hard to check for small samples. Parametric methods like the t-test or analysis of variance cannot be used without a suitable transformation as the data are markedly non-normal. Other methods assume a Poisson (Amphlett and Delow, 1984; Brodin, 1989) or a negative binomial (Mackey and MacGregor, 1979) distribution.

Tests which assume the cell to be the experimental unit instead of the animal are inappropriate, e.g., Fisher's exact test, the χ^2-test (Hart and Engberg-Pedersen, 1983) and the test of Kastenbaum and Bowman (1970).

Non-parametric methods such as the Kruskal-Wallis test use the rank information only (PSI, 1986). Small sample sizes and ties are a problem if these tests are not performed using the exact distribution. The Kolmogorov-Smirnov test, suggested by Mitchell and Brice (1986), has lower power in comparison to several other methods (Lovell and Fellows, 1987).
Williams (1988) suggested permutation tests for the analysis of small, simply-structured data sets arising from toxicological experiments. The permutation method does not rely on distributional assumptions or asymptotic distributions of the test statistics. In the present paper the Fisher-Pitman permutation test (Lehmann, 1975) is proposed for the statistical analysis of the micronucleus test.

Method

In the Fisher-Pitman test, two independent samples of size N_1 and N_2 are compared with respect to location. The difference between the means is used as the test statistic. The p-value of the one-sided test is calculated using the permutation technique:
First the difference between the observed means in the two samples is determined. Then the $r = \binom{N_1 + N_2}{N_1}$ different partitions of the $N_1 + N_2$ observations into artificial samples of size N_1 and N_2, respectively, are formed. For each partition there is a value of the difference between the means. Under the null hypothesis "no location shift", all these differences are equally likely. Let k be the number of partitions, in which the difference of the means is greater or equal to the observed difference. The p-value of the one-sided Fisher-Pitman test is then calculated as $p = k/r$. The null hypothesis is rejected if p is less than the chosen level of significance.

Example

One of the typical designs of the mouse bone marrow micronucleus test includes a negative (vehicle) control group, a positive control group and three identically treated groups which are analyzed at different times (24 h, 48 h and 72 h after administration of the test substance). For both sexes each treatment group is compared with the negative control group. The p-values of the one-sided Fisher-Pitman test are reported.

Table 1. Number of micronucleated polychromatic erythrocytes (MPE) per 2000 polychromatic erythrocytes assessed per animal with the p-values of the one-sided Fisher-Pitman test for comparison with the negative control group (5 animals per group)

Sampling point	Number of MPE		p-value
	Individual counts	Mean	
Males:			
Negative control	3, 4, 2, 4, 3	3.2	
Test substance:			
24 h after administration	2, 9, 7, 1, 7	5.2	0.131
48 h after administration	10, 4, 9, 10, 9	8.4	0.012
72 h after administration	9, 3, 7, 2, 4	5.0	0.175
Positive control	24, 18, 22, 31, 27	24.4	0.004
Females:			
Negative control	7, 2, 9, 1, 2	4.2	
Test substance:			
24 h after administration	5, 5, 8, 5, 7	6.0	0.187
48 h after administration	7, 5, 5, 10, 6	6.6	0.139
72 h after administration	5, 5, 11, 2, 4	5.4	0.337
Positive control	33, 19, 29, 24, 31	27.2	0.004

For the data in Table 1, the number of micronucleated polychromatic erythrocytes of the males at 48 h is at the 5%-level significantly higher than in the negative control group. The same holds for the positive control groups of both sexes.
No adjustment for multiple testing is performed as the three sampling points were chosen because test substances differ in the time after treatment at which the peak frequency of micronuclei occurs.

Discussion

The Fisher-Pitman test is recommended as a suitable method for evaluating the micronucleus test. It takes into account the characteristics of the micronucleus test (the animal is the experimental unit, the data consist of integer counts with ties, the sample sizes are small). It avoids the specification of a distribution for the number of micronucleated polychromatic erythrocytes and uses the observed data without transformation.
With modern computers it is no longer a problem to calculate the distribution of a permutation test statistic. Algorithms are available which make it possible to compute the p-value of the Fisher-Pitman test on a PC (Streitberg and Röhmel, 1986; Voß, 1989).

References

Amphlett GE, Delow GF (1984). Statistical analysis of the micronucleus test. Mutation Research, 128, 161-166 .

Brodin U (1989). Statistical analysis of the micronucleus test - a modelling approach. Mutation Research, 211, 259-264 .

Hart JW, Engberg-Pedersen H (1983). Statistics of the mouse bone-marrow micronucleus test: counting, distribution and evaluation of results. Mutation Research, 111, 195-207.

Kastenbaum MA, Bowman KO (1970). Tables for determining the statistical significance of mutation frequencies. Mutation Research, 9, 527-549 .

Kirkland DJ (Ed.) (1989). Statistical Evaluation of Mutagenicity Test Data. Cambridge University Press, Cambridge.

Lehmann EL (1975). Nonparametrics. Holden-Day, Oakland, California.

Lovell DP, Fellows DM (1987). A comparison of statistical methods for the analysis of micronucleus assay data using a computer simulation study. Mutagenesis, 2, 311 .

MacGregor JT, Heddle JA, Hite M, Margolin BH, Ramel C, Salome MF, Tice RR, Wild D (1987). Guidelines for the conduct of micronucleus assays in mammalian bone marrow erythrocytes. Mutation Research, 189, 103-112.

Mackey BE, MacGregor JT (1979). The micronucleus test: Statistical design and analysis. Mutation Research, 64, 195-204 .

Mitchell I de G, Brice AJ (1986). Investigations into parametric analysis of data from in vivo micronucleus assays by comparison with non-parametric methods. Mutation Research, 159, 139-146 .

PSI (1986). Report of PSI working party on the data produced by the ABPI collaborative study into the micronucleus test. Unpublished report.

Schmid W (1975). The micronuleus test. Mutation Research, 31, 9-15 .

Streitberg B, Röhmel J (1986). Exact distributions for permutation and rank tests: an introduction to some recently published algorithms. Statist. Software Newsletter, 12, 10-17 .

Voß H (1989). Exact distribution for 2-sample-permutation and rank-tests using the Streitberg-Röhmel-Algorithm and SAS/IML Software. Proceedings of the SAS European Users Group International Conference, Cologne, 28-37 .

Williams DA (1988). Extra-binomial variation in toxicology. Proceedings of the XIVth International Biometric Conference, Namur, 301-313 .

A STATISTICAL ANALYSIS OF HGPRT–TEST DATA BY MEANS OF COMPUTER SIMULATIONS

Stefan Rettig
Zentrum für Praktische Mathematik, Technische Hochschule Darmstadt
Hochschulstraße 1, 6100 Darmstadt

Jürgen Lehn
Fachbereich Mathematik, Technische Hochschule Darmstadt
Schloßgartenstraße 7, 6100 Darmstadt

Herbert G. Miltenburger
Laboratorium für Mutagenitätsprüfung, Technische Hochschule Darmstadt
Schnittspahnstraße 3, 6100 Darmstadt

1 Introduction

The Chemical Act first issued by the Federal Government of Germany in 1980 includes regulations in order to prevent mutagenic chemicals from becoming a risk for the population. Producers and distributors of chemicals must present data from mutagenicity tests showing that there is no measurable mutagenic potential. The Laboratory for Mutagenicity Testing (Laboratorium für Mutagenitätsprüfung = LMP) is routinely performing such tests for state administrations and industry under contract.

For the evaluation of the mutagenic potential of chemicals data from both in vitro and in vivo tests have to be elaborated. Quite often in vitro tests with bacteria (e. g. Ames–test) and mammalian cell cultures (e. g. chromosome aberration test) are applied first. If the results from these tests require further testing, in vivo assays are usually performed. However, whenever experiments with animals can be avoided, in vitro test systems should be used with priority.

It is the aim of our interdisciplinary research work to contribute to the improvement of in vitro methods by including relevant biometrical methods which help effectively to decide whether a chemical must be classified as mutagenic or not. Such decisions are generally difficult and subjective in the case when data from experiments are obtained in the range between clear negative and clear positive findings.

2 The formulation of the problem

The most frequently used in vitro mutation assay is the Salmonella typhimurium/liver microsome test, named AMES–test after Dr. B. N. Ames who developed it. The test measures reversion events in mutated strains of S. typhimurium. For the detection of gene mutations in vitro the HGPRT–test–system with cultures of mammalian cells (V79- or CHO–cells; Chinese Hamster origin) is commonly used. Because of the world wide acceptance of this test system and its high degree of interlaboratory standardization we thought it would be worthwhile investigating the correlation of mutation data and statistics.

HGPRT (hypoxanthine–guanine–phosphoribosyl–transferase) is an enzyme which is produced by normal cells. However, a cell can loose the ability to produce this enzyme by a gene mutation either spontaneously or by induction. Such mutations can be recognized when cell clones from mutant cells are formed in a special selective medium. Non–mutants die in this medium. The mutant colonies are stained and counted at the end of the test.

The evaluation of data from a HGPRT–test is influenced by spontaneously occuring mutations which appear in an absolute random way. For this reason untreated control groups are run in parallel to the cell cultures treated with the test chemical. The mutation frequency observed in such "negative" controls and its variability is important for the decision whether a chemical significantly induces mutations leading to a higher frequency as compared to the negative (= spontaneous) mutation frequency.

Appropriate statistical analyses of test data are recommended by international guidelines. Of course this recommendation applies also for the performance of the HGPRT–test according to guidelines published by the EEC (European Economic Community), the OECD (Organization for Economic Co–Operation and Development), the American organizations EPA (Environmental Protection Agency) and FDA (Food and Drug Administration). However, there are no adequate and satisfactory proposals of how these requirements could be fulfilled. Two proposals, one given by Irr et al. (1979) and Snee et al. (1981) and another by Hsie et al. (1975) and Arlett et al. (1989) did not solve the problem. The methods used in these studies are based on the mutant frequencies observed at the end of the test. They did not consider specific properties of the HGPRT–system on one hand and the fact that the special experimental design may vary from laboratory to laboratory on the other hand. Decisions of whether a chemical has to be considered mutagenic or not are often influenced by subjective interpretations for the lack of adequate and appropriate statistical methods. Therefore, we undertook the studies presented in the following on the basis of a detailed analysis of the quality of a special experimental design which is thought to contribute to an improvement of the statistical treatment of experimental results thus reducing the probability of the risk of incorrect classifications in mutagenicity testing. The research aims are the following:

- To specify a statistical evaluation method given as an "evaluation formula" where the parameters of the experimental design and the properties of the cells are taken into account together with the observed mutation frequencies.

- To develop methods which allow to foresee how changes in the experimental design affect the amount of information in the final evaluation.

- To provide tools which can be used to perform a quality comparison of different experimental designs and different "evaluation formulae".

3 Methods

In order to accomplish these tasks, a mathematical model has been developed for the biological processes and the experimental handling according to the experimental design. For each data determination the measuring error has been described by a random variable, for each subculturing step a random variable has been introduced which characterizes the randomly varying number of the spontaneous mutants seeded in the subculture, etc. Especially the following problems had to be solved:

- A mathematical description had to be worked out for the effects of mutagenicity and toxicity of the test compound. Eckardt and Haynes (1979, 1980, 1981, 1985) developed such a model based on the same ideas as the hit models for the X–ray treatment of cells. This model could be modified for the biochemical processes during treatment to describe them in a sufficiently exact way.

- A mathematical description had to be found for the cell multiplication and proliferation of cell population and the resulting increase of the spontaneous mutation frequency. This has been done by a Markov chain model which in particular takes into account the reduction of the concentration of the HGPRT enzyme in the cells after a mutation (see Rettig (1990)).

- The plating of cells and the determination of the plating efficiency had to be modelled. A hierarchical model can be used as description of the actual plating process. The effects of the experimental handling which has to be performed according to the experimental design are characterized by a system of conditional distributions (see Rettig (1990)).

All other biochemical and technical processes during the performance of the HGPRT–test are affected without exception by randomness and random measurement errors. They have been described by numerous dependent random variables. Altogether the elaborated stochastic model contains approximately 7000 different random variables corresponding to biochemical processes or experimental handling steps. This enormous number of variables is not astonishing if one thinks of the performance of the HGPRT–test which takes about three weeks and needs a lot of experimental handling. About 30 treatment and control groups (negative and positive) are involved and have to be modelled separately (see the experimental design of the HGPRT–test in the Laboratory for Mutagenicity Testing at Darmstadt University of Technology in Figure 1).

The stochastic model yet contains a number of free parameters as e. g. the time of a cell cycle and the plating efficiency of cells which have to be adjusted very carefully. This problem of data fitting has been solved together with the mathematical modelling. A data base has been built up for this purpose at the Centre for Applied Mathematics consisting in the data from HGPRT–tests performed in the Laboratory for Mutagenicity Testing during the past five years. These approximately 80000 data give very precise information about

1st day (wed): thawing
cell growth 48 h
3rd day (fri): subculturing
cell growth 72 h
6th day (mon): seeding exp. 1
cell growth 48 h
8th day (wed): seeding exp. 2
cell growth 24 h
7th day (tue): treatment exp. 1
cell growth 72 h
10th day (fri): subculturing exp. 1
cell growth 96 h
14th day (tue): selection exp. 1
cell growth (cell death of non mutants) 192 h
22th day (wed): staining exp. 1
cell growth 24 h
9th day (thu): treatment exp. 2
cell growth 96 h
13th day (mon): subculturing exp. 2
cell growth 72 h
16th day (thu): selection exp. 2
cell growth (cell death of non mutants) 192 h
24th day (fri): staining exp. 2

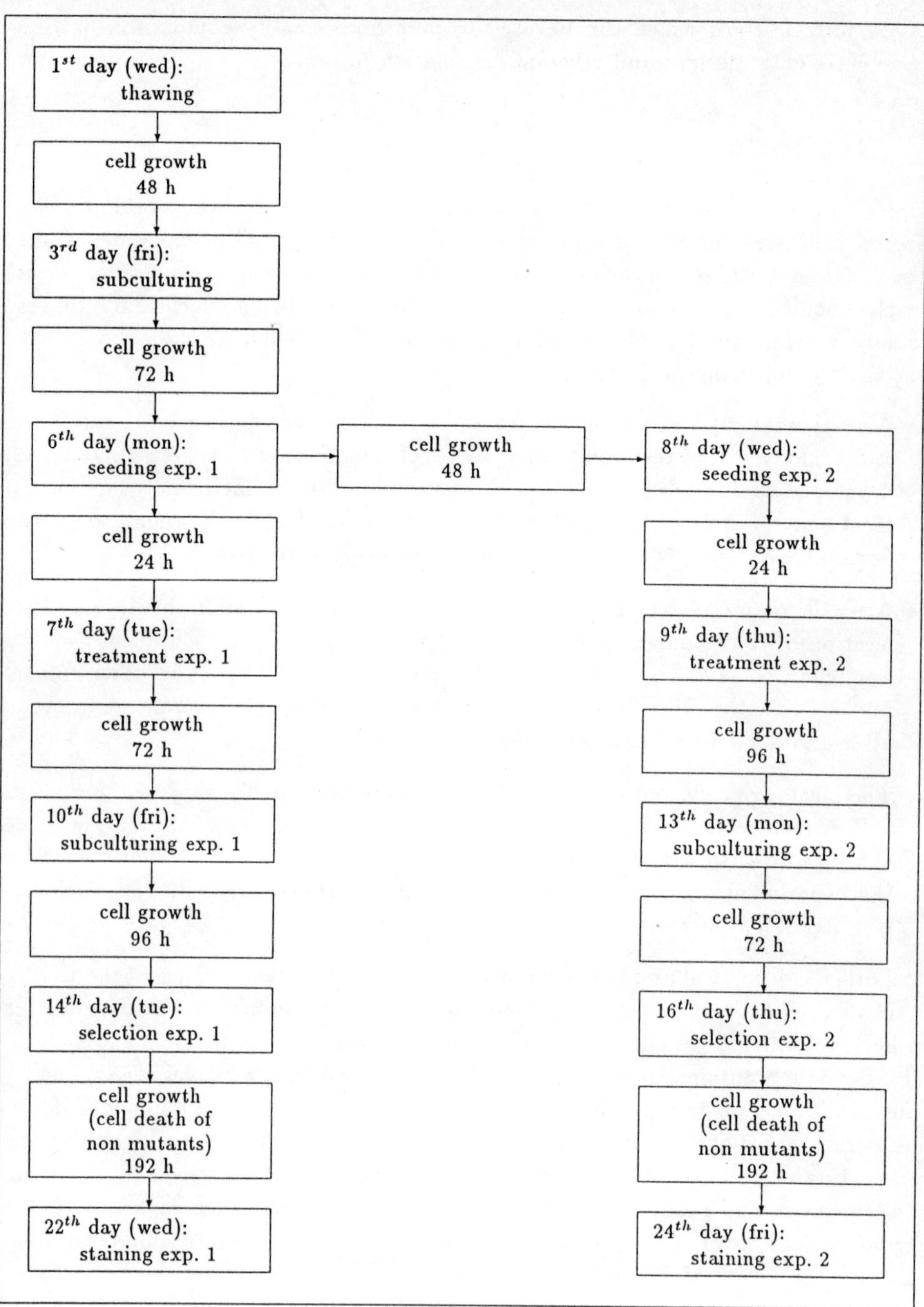

Figure 1

the values of the free parameters in the model when they are analysed with appropriate statistical methods. For each parameter estimation appropriate estimators had to be chosen so that the information about the parameter contained in the data base could be exploited in an efficient way.

A comprehensive mathematical analysis has been made by mathematicians and biologists in cooperation on the whole biological test system. Not only subproblems have been solved as it has been done in many other mathematical investigations in the field of mutagenicity testing. The intention was to model the complete mutagenicity assay such that practical questions could be answered by means of computer simulations. Originally it was planned to incorporate the results of W. Y. Tan (1983, 1989) on branching processes for modelling the cell growth. This was rejected because the complexity of these methods would have needed huge CPU times for one single simulation within the whole test performance.

4 The evaluation process

The problem of the statistical evaluation of the test results has still to be solved after modelling the whole test system and after adjusting the model through estimation of the free model parameters with help of the data from the data base. The issue was to formulate the mathematical problem in such a way that it could be analysed with the methods and concepts of mathematical statistics. The first step was to introduce a "mutagenicity parameter" θ which describes the mutagenic activity of a chemical. This parameter corresponds to the increase of the mutation frequency caused by the test compound during the performance of the HGPRT–test, or more precisely:

> θ is the number of mutants induced by the test compound per 10^6 cells (referred to a certain unit dose)

Therefore, the test problem which corresponds to the evaluation of the HGPRT–test data is the decision between the null hypothesis

$$H_0 \;:\quad \theta = 0 \qquad \text{"non mutagenic chemical"}$$

and the alternative

$$H_1 \;:\quad \theta > 0 \qquad \text{"mutagenic chemical"}$$

where, of course, "non mutagenic" only means that no mutations occur at the HGPRT gene locus. A test statistic

$$T(y_1, \ldots, y_c; x_1, \ldots, x_t)$$

is suggested to be applied for solving this decision problem which depends on the corrected (according to the experimental design) mutant frequencies $y_1, \ldots, y_c$ in the control groups and on the mutant frequencies $x_1, \ldots, x_t$, also corrected, in the treatment groups. If the case $c = 4$ and $t = 8$ is considered, then the test statistic is given by the formula

$$T(y_1, \ldots, y_4; x_1, \ldots, x_8) =$$
$$\sum_{i=1}^{4} \frac{-1}{8d_i} \cdot \ln\left[1 - \frac{x_i - \frac{1}{2}(y_1 + y_2)}{1 - \frac{1}{2}(y_1 + y_2)}\right] + \sum_{i=5}^{8} \frac{-1}{8d_{i-4}} \cdot \ln\left[1 - \frac{x_i - \frac{1}{2}(y_3 + y_4)}{1 - \frac{1}{2}(y_3 + y_4)}\right]$$

where the y–values and the x–values correspond with the corrected results in the control groups and in the treatment groups, respectively, $y_1, y_2, x_1, \ldots, x_4$ are the corrected results in experiment 1, $y_3, y_4, x_5, \ldots, x_8$ are the corrected results in experiment 2, and $d_1, \ldots, d_4$ are the doses of the 4 treatment groups in both experiments. The form of this test statistic is derived from the model for the effects of mutagenicity and toxicity. In this model a linear dose–response pattern is used to describe the effects of mutagenicity and a quadratic–cubic dose–response pattern to characterize the effects of toxicity. A linearization of the logarithm terms leads to the following more lucid formula which gives approximately the same values

$$T(y_1, \ldots, y_4; x_1, \ldots, x_8) \approx \sum_{i=1}^{4} \frac{x_i - \frac{1}{2}(y_1 + y_2)}{8d_i} + \sum_{i=5}^{8} \frac{x_i - \frac{1}{2}(y_3 + y_4)}{8d_{i-4}}$$

The correction of the observed data is derived from the Markov chain model for the cell growth during the whole test performance. The correction formulae are omitted here and can be found in Rettig (1990). Simulation studies show immediately that this is an appropriate test statistic for the decision problem at hand: The distribution of the test statistic shifts towards growing T–values with growing θ (see Figure 2).

With this test statistic the path of classical test theory has been followed: For a given significance level α, e. g. $\alpha = 0.05$, a threshold c_α has been determined by simulation which is exceeded by the test statistic with probability α under the null hypothesis H_0. This has been done by applying a suitable quantile estimator to the simulation results. The test statistic T and the threshold c_α define a statistical decision rule by which the chemical has to be classified as follows:

$$\begin{array}{lcl} T > c_\alpha & : & \text{mutagenic} \\ T \le c_\alpha & : & \text{non mutagenic} \end{array}$$

Because of its construction this is a decision rule where the probability of a type I error equals α or more precisely, it approximately equals α since the threshold c_α cannot be calculated and has to be determined by means of simulation. Recall, a type I error occurs if a non mutagenic test compound (i. e. $\theta = 0$) is misclassified as mutagenic.

Other proposals for such α-level decision rules have already been made (see Arlett et al. (1989), Hsie et al. (1975), Irr et al. (1979), Snee et al. (1981)). They are based on less substantiated and less convincing test statistics since they are chosen independently of the biological context. Nevertheless,

> the probability for classifying a non mutagenic chemical as mutagenic is approximately equal to α.

This type I error which may occur when HGPRT–test data are evaluated has to be taken into consideration but the type II error, i. e. the misclassification of a mutagenic chemical, is the much more serious one. Therefore,

> the probability of classifying a mutagenic chemical as non mutagenic

is much more important.

mutation frequency at the beginning = 0,00
spontaneous mutation rate = 8,00*10^-7
number of control groups per exp. = 2
number of treatment groups per exp. = 4
number of simulation runs = 500
k2 = 1,5*10^-3
k3 = 5,2*10^-8
θ = 0,0
m = 0,03
s = 0,55
relative frequency [%]
value of test statistic (×10^-6)
20,0
18,0
16,0
14,0
12,0
10,0
8,0
6,0
4,0
2,0
0,0
-3,0
-2,0
-1,0
0,0
1,0
2,0
3,0
4,0
5,0

mutation frequency at the beginning = 0,00
spontaneous mutation rate = 8,00*10^-7
number of control groups per exp. = 2
number of treatment groups per exp. = 4
number of simulation runs = 500
k2 = 1,5*10^-3
k3 = 5,2*10^-8
θ = 2,0*10^-6
m = 2,01
s = 0,63
relative frequency [%]
value of test statistic (×10^-6)
20,0
18,0
16,0
14,0
12,0
10,0
8,0
6,0
4,0
2,0
0,0
-3,0
-2,0
-1,0
0,0
1,0
2,0
3,0
4,0
5,0

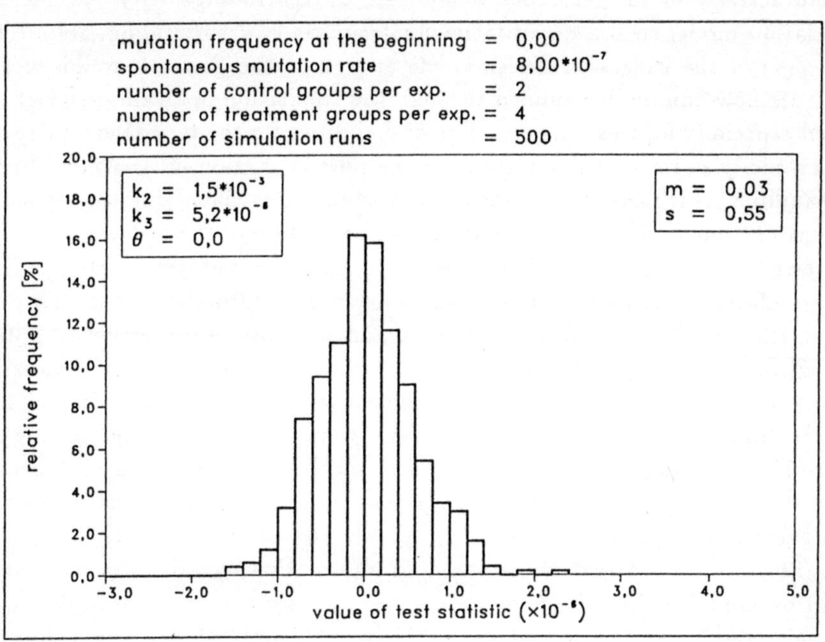

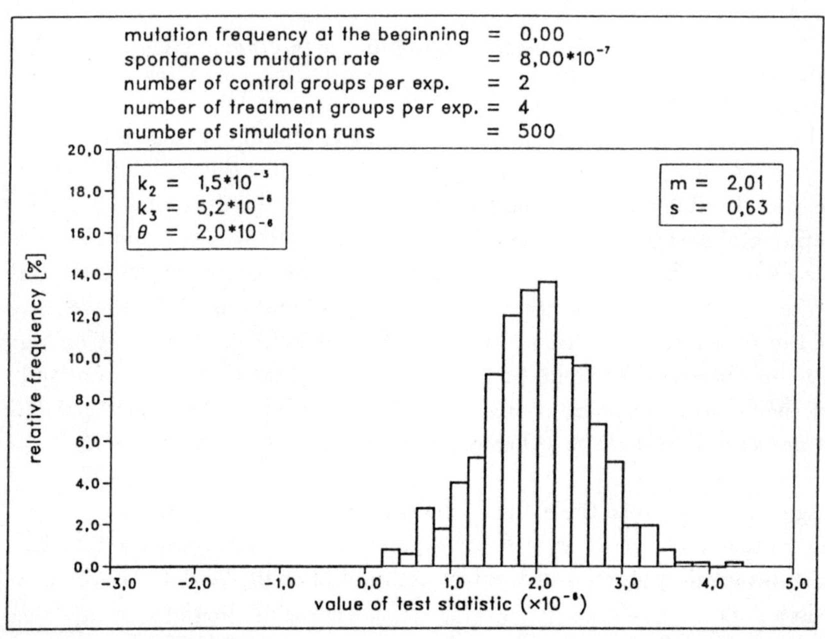

Figure 2

This probability could not be quantified so far and it depends, of course, on the mutagenic activity of the test compound, i.e. on the mutagenicity parameter θ. By the simulation model such a quantitative analysis has now become possible. The power function $g(\theta)$ of the suggested decision rule as well as the power function of any other decision rule now can be determined through the simulation programme which has been developed especially for this purpose. The probabilities for the type II error depending on the mutagenicity parameter θ are given by the power function $g(\theta)$. Above all these are the probabilities which have to be taken into account when classifying the test compound. The laboratory personnel responsible for the classification of the test compound must be able to refer to these error probabilities when judging the mutagenic activity.

The simulation programme supplies this important information. It is now possible to determine the efficiency of the HGPRT–test and to study the question of optimal test design and the optimality of the statistical decision rule to be applied for classifying the test compound. Today it is quite easy to recognize a clearly mutagenic chemical. It is much more difficult to detect a weakly mutagenic chemical by established testing methods. Therefore it is very important to analyse these methods in the "weak mutagenic range" and to increase their sensitivity by varying the experimental design as well as the statistical decision rule to be applied to the data. Proposals are made for such changes (see Rettig (1990)). So it turns out that the amount of information contained in the data can be increased by minimal changes of the dose levels used for the treatment groups, i. e. the risk of a misclassification can be reduced in this way. Figure 3 shows three power functions $g(\theta)$ for different combinations of dose levels when the decision rule described above

"classify the test compound as mutagenic if
$T(y_1, \ldots, y_c; x_1, \ldots, x_t) > c_\alpha$ "

is applied to the simulated data. The figures refer to the significance level $\alpha = 0.05$. The steeper the slope of the power function $g(\theta)$ is, the smaller the probabilities for a type II error are, i. e. the higher the amount of information in the data of a HGPRT–test with this experimental design is. The second figure corresponds to a combination of dose levels which are chosen according to the requirements in the official guidelines. But it turns out (see the first picture in Figure 3) that other combinations of dose levels give steeper slopes of the power function $g(\theta)$, i. e. a HGPRT–test with these dose combinations is more efficient. However, it should be mentioned again that this simulation study is based upon two special dose–response patterns for the mutagenic and toxic effects. Other dose–response patterns may lead to other recommendations for changes in the experimental design.

The figures contain also the value θ_β defined by $g(\theta_\beta) = 1 - \beta$ for $\beta = 0.05$. The value θ_β of the mutagenicity parameter θ corresponds to the mutagenicity threshold beyond which the mutagenic potential of the test compound could be detected with probability greater than 0.95.

In the same way different decision rules can be compared by means of the simulation programme developed in the Centre for Applied Mathematics at Darmstadt University of Technology. Because of the flexible structure of this computer programme it is possible to simulate experimental designs of the HGPRT–test which may or may not differ from

mutation frequency at the beginning = 5,00*10
spontaneous mutation rate = 8,00*10
number of control groups per exp. = 2
number of treatment groups per exp. = 4
β = 0,05
θ_β = 1,23
k₂ = 1,5*10
k₃ = 5,2*10
α = 0,05
c_α = 0,56
power function g(θ)
mutagenicity parameter θ
dose 1 : LD10
dose 2 : LD25
dose 3 : LD40
dose 4 : LD60
mutation frequency at the beginning = 5,00*10
spontaneous mutation rate = 8,00*10
number of control groups per exp. = 2
number of treatment groups per exp. = 4
β = 0,05
θ_β = 2,48
k₂ = 1,5*10
k₃ = 5,2*10
α = 0,05
c_α = 1,18
power function g(θ)
mutagenicity parameter θ
dose 1 : LD01
dose 2 : LD20
dose 3 : LD50
dose 4 : LD80
mutation frequency at the beginning = 5,00*10
spontaneous mutation rate = 8,00*10
number of control groups per exp. = 2
number of treatment groups per exp. = 4
β = 0,05
θ_β = 3,09
k₂ = 1,5*10
k₃ = 5,2*10
α = 0,05
c_α = 1,39
power function g(θ)
mutagenicity parameter θ
dose 1 : LD01
dose 2 : LD05
dose 3 : LD15
dose 4 : LD20

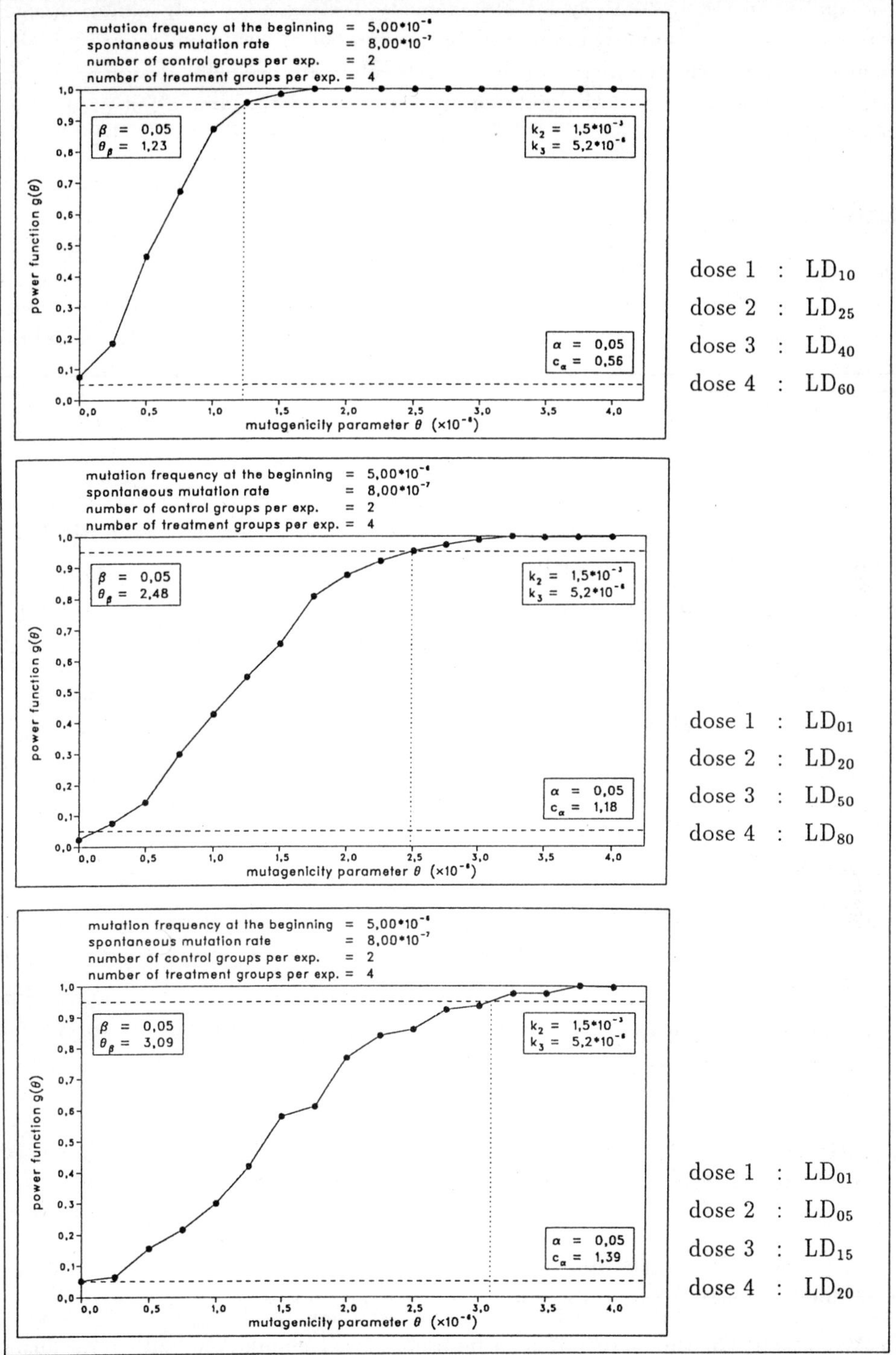

Figure 3

those applied in the Laboratory for Mutagenicity Testing, i. e. only minor changes of the input parameters (number of control groups, number of treatment groups, number of subculturing steps, characteristics of the cell line, etc.) are needed.

A detailed description of the mathematical model and the simulation programme is given by Rettig (1990).

References

Arlett, CF, Smith, DM, Green, MHL, McGregor, DB, Clarke, GM, Cole, J, Asquith, JC (1989) Mammalian cell gene mutation assays based upon colony formation. in: Kirkland, DJ (1989) Statistical evaluation of mutagenicity test data. Cambridge, New York, Port Chester, Melbourne, Sidney: Cambridge University Press, 66–101

Eckardt, F, Haynes, RH (1979) Mathematical analysis of mutation–induction kinetics. Genet. Cytol. 21: 271–302

Eckardt, F, Haynes, RH (1981) Quantitative measures of induced mutagenesis. in: Stich, HF, San, RHC (1981) Short–term tests for chemical carcinogens. Berlin, Heidelberg, New York: Springer Verlag, 457–473

Eckardt, F, Haynes, RH (1980) Quantitative measures of mutagenicity and mutability based on mutant yield data. Mutation Research 74: 439–458

Haynes, RH, Eckardt, F, Kunz, BA (1985) Analysis of non–linearities in mutation frequency curves. Mutation Research 150: 51–59

Hsie, AW, Brimer, PA, Mitchell, TJ, Gosslee, DG (1975) The dose–response relationship for ethyl methanesulfonate–induced mutations at the hypoxanthin–guanine phosphoribosyl transferase locus in Chinese hamster ovary cells. Somatic Cell Genetics 1: 247–261

Irr, JD, Snee, RD (1979) Statistical evaluation of mutagenicity in the CHO/HGPRT–system. Mammalian cell mutagenesis: The mutation test system. Banbury Report 2: 263–275

Rettig, S (1990) Modellierung, Simulation und statistische Analyse des HGPRT–Mutagenitätstests. Dissertation, Fachbereich Mathematik, Technische Hochschule Darmstadt

Snee, RD, Irr, JD (1981) Design of a statistical method for the analysis of mutagenesis at the HGPRT–locus of cultured chinese hamster ovary cells. Mutation Research 85: 77–93

Tan, WY (1983) On the distribution of the number of mutants at the HGPRT–locus in Chinese hamster ovary cells. Math. Biosci. 67: 175–192

Tan, WY (1989) On the distribution of mutants in cell populations with both forward and backward mutation. Siam. J. Appl. Math. 49: 186–196

MEASURING INTRA-ASSAY AGREEMENT FOR THE AMES *SALMONELLA* ASSAY

Walter W. Piegorsch and Errol Zeiger
National Institute of Environmental Health Sciences,
Research Triangle Park, NC 27709, USA

Introduction

To assess the effects of exposure to toxic stimuli, the U.S. National Toxicology Program (NTP) conducts bioassays in various organisms, each with a different biological endpoint. Mutagenic damage, as indicated by the *Salmonella* assay (Ames et al., 1975), is a major concern. The *Salmonella* assay occupies a central role in the genotoxicity testing program undertaken by the NTP. This program has involved numerous chemicals, tested under code, and under strictly controlled protocols at a number of laboratories.

The accumulated NTP *Salmonella* database has been examined to assess the qualitative reproducibility of results from the assay (Dunkel et al., 1984; 1985). It was found that the qualitative reproducibility among laboratories for a given chemical was generally good, but no descriptive or inferential biometric techniques were employed to quantify the degree of this agreement. Such quantifications are of clear interest, and are performed herein.

Database Construction

The database of interest derives from NTP assays for *Salmonella* mutagenicity. Portions of the data from these assays are summarized by Haworth et al. (1983), Mortelmans et al. (1986), and Zeiger et al. (1987; 1988). Selected chemicals were tested more than once in the same, or different, laboratories, at different times over an eight-year period. Each time a chemical was tested, it was sent to the testing laboratory under a different chemical code number, so that the laboratory was unaware of the chemical's previous testing. Specific details regarding the tester strains, assay protocol, and per-assay evaluations may be found in Zeiger et al. (1987; 1988).

The *Salmonella* assay, as performed by the NTP, results in one of four qualitative conclusions as to the evidence for mutagenicity: Positive (+), Weak Positive (+W), Negative (-), or Questionable/Equivocal (?). The agreement across these four qualitative categories was examined by appealing to the results from all chemicals subject to repeat testing by the NTP, with results reported and cleared as of 1 August 1988. This database has 239 chemicals, as presented in Table 1.

Statistical Measures: Descriptive

Denote by X_{ij} the number of observed conclusions for the ith chemical in the jth conclusion category (i=1,...,N; j=1,...,k). For the NTP data, N=239 and j=1,...,4 (i.e., k=4) corresponding to j=+,+W,-,?. The number of conclusions attained (i.e., different samples tested) for the ith chemical is denoted by m_i, so that $\sum_{i=1}^{4} X_{ij} = m_i$.

The various chemicals in Table 1 were not always retested in a balanced fashion; i.e., the values of m_i exhibited in Table 1 are generally 2, but further retests can drive this as high as 12. This imbalance is not purely random: certain chemicals are of greater importance and interest, and are retested more often. The effect of this imbalance on the statistical measures is noted below.

The statistical methods employed to assess quantitatively the level of agreement displayed in the NTP database involves both descriptive and inferential components. For the purely descriptive statistics, each chemical provides a measure of concordance across conclusion categories: perfect agreement corresponds to perfect concordance, where only one category displays a non-zero entry. Such perfect across-category concordance is assigned a per-chemical concordance of '1'. Any deviation from this perfect across-category concordance is strictly interpreted as a discordance, to which a per-chemical concordance of '0' is assigned. The observed average of these per-chemical concordances serves as a summary measure of overall agreement. This strict measure of concordance corresponds to that employed by Gold et al. (1987) in their study of "near-replicate" assay results for rodent carcinogenicity. If m_i=2, it corresponds to simple percentage concordance, described and examined, e.g., by Kupper and Hafner (1989, eq. 2).

Such strict per-chemical concordance is a very conservative measure of agreement. Clearly, a chemical tested 12 times with, say, 11 positive responses and 1 negative response exhibits a higher degree of agreement than one tested only twice with 1 positive and 1 negative response. Nevertheless, the strict measure described above assigns a zero concordance to both chemicals. To alleviate this conservatism, a concordance measure that attempts to quantify the amount of *pairwise* agreement among multiple inter-sample/intra-chemical responses can also be derived. For every possible pair of outcomes for a given chemical, count the number of pairs exhibiting concordance. Then, divide this number by the total number of possible pairs for that chemical. The pairwise agreement is then simply $[\sum_{j=1}^{4} X_{ij}(X_{ij}-1)]/m_i(m_i-1)$. This scheme inherently corrects for differences in numbers of responses (i.e., differing m_i) via the pairing mechanism. Returning to the examples above, a response of X_{i1}=11, X_{i3}=1, X_{i2}=X_{i4}=0 (11+, 1-) gives 55 possible concordant pairs, out of a total of 66 possible pairs. The corresponding observed pairwise concordance is $\frac{55}{66}$ = 83.33% rather than the zero given by the strict measure, above. A response of $X_{i'1}$=$X_{i'3}$=1, $X_{i'2}$=$X_{i'4}$=0 (1+,1-), however, shows no concordant pairs out of one possible pair. Thus its pairwise concordance agrees with the strict result of zero. Indeed, for those chemicals where m_i=2, the pairwise and strict concordances must always agree.

These two calculated concordance measures are separately averaged over all chemicals to yield summary concordances. These summaries values are descriptive measures of percentage agreement.

Statistical Measures: Inferential

It should be noted that any simple measure of qualitative agreement such as average concordance may be observed at high levels *purely by chance*. That is, the true underlying concordance may be very close to zero, but by chance alone the observed concordance may be observed to approach one (a sort of "false positive" indication). For qualitative categorizations, a chance-corrected measure of agreement is the Kappa coefficient, κ (Cohen, 1960). Denoting the proportion of agreement expected by chance alone as P_e, and the overall percentage agreement by P_o, the proportion of agreement attributable to underlying reproducibility after correcting for chance agreement is $\kappa = (P_o - P_e)/(1 - P_e)$ (Gross, 1986). This value varies from -1 to +1. At κ=+1, perfect agreement is indicated, while at κ=-1, perfect disagreement is indicated. At κ=0, no deviation from purely chance agreement is evidenced. For the problem of multiple categories, such as the four categories described herein, one can apply Gross' (1986) extension of κ, which includes a maximum likelihood estimator, $\hat{\kappa}$, for the true underlying agreement.

To calculate Gross' estimate of κ, one begins with the raw sample proportions of categorical agreement: $T_{ij} = X_{ij}/m_i$ and $\overline{T}_j = \Sigma_{i=1}^{N} m_i T_{ij}/M$, with $M = \Sigma_{i=1}^{N} m_i$. Then, one has

$$\hat{\kappa} = \sum_{i=1}^{N} \sum_{j=1}^{k} \frac{m_i (T_{ij} - \overline{T}_j)^2}{M \overline{T}_j (k-1)} \quad .$$

A large-sample variance estimator for $\hat{\kappa}$ is (Gross, 1986)

$$\widehat{\mathrm{var}}(\hat{\kappa}) = \frac{\sum_{i=1}^{N} m_i \left\{ \sum_{j=1}^{k} T_{ij} g_{ij}^2 - \left(\sum_{j=1}^{k} T_{ij} g_{ij} \right)^2 \right\}}{[M(k-1)]^2}$$

where $g_{ij} = 2T_{ij}(1-m_i/M)/T_{ij} - \Sigma_{i=1}^{N} m_i(T_{ij}-T_j)^2/(MT_j)^2$. Gross' measure is designed to correct for possible imbalance among the m_i, and retains its asymptotic characteristics — such as large-sample normality for $\hat{\kappa}$ — no matter what pattern of m_i's is observed.

Results

Application of the measures of agreement presented above to the 239-chemical NTP database yields:

Strict concordance	Pairwise concordance	$\hat{\kappa}$	95% confidence limits
$\frac{161}{239} = 67.36\%$	71.46%	0.631	(0.575 , 0.686)

The inference available from the κ-analysis implies that agreement in the data differs significantly from zero, and is, indeed, strongly positive even after correcting for any chance agreement. Collapsing the + and +W categories into one "positive" category gives similar results:

Strict concordance	Pairwise concordance	$\hat{\kappa}$	95% confidence limits
$\frac{169}{239} = 70.71\%$	74.48%	0.653	(0.573 , 0.733)

Removing the Equivocal category from the database, but retaining the + and +W distinction, leaves outcomes from 206 chemicals for comparison (losses occur from chemicals with no or only one total outcome in the non-equivocal categories). For these (non-equivocal) data:

Strict concordance	Pairwise concordance	$\hat{\kappa}$	95% confidence limits
$\frac{163}{206} = 79.13\%$	83.22%	0.730	(0.679 , 0.780)

Collapsing the + and +W categories further, as performed above, leads to a two-category comparison: "any Positive" vs. Negative:

Strict concordance	Pairwise concordance	$\hat{\kappa}$	95% confidence limits
$\frac{174}{206} = 84.47\%$	86.89%	0.861	(0.843 , 0.880)

The level of intra-assay agreement for *Salmonella* mutagenicity evidenced in the NTP database is quite good. Descriptive measures yield percentage concordances between roughly 70% and 90%. Formal statistical analyses of the (chance-corrected) level of agreement are all strongly significant. These conclusions remain valid under various pertinent sub-divisions and sub-groupings of the data.

References

Ames BN, McCann J, Yamasaki E (1975) Methods for detecting carcinogens and mutagens with the *Salmonella*/mammalian microsome mutagenicity test. Mutat. Res. 31:347-364.

Cohen J (1960) A coefficient of agreement for nominal scales. Psych. Bull. 70:213-220.

Dunkel VC, Zeiger E, Brusick D, McCoy E, McGregor D, Mortelmans K, Rosenkranz HS, Simmon VF (1984) Reproducibility of microbial mutagenicity assays: I. Tests with *Salmonella typhimurium* and *Escherichia coli* using a standardized protocol. Environ. Mutagen. 6 (suppl. 2):1-251.

Dunkel VC, Zeiger E, Brusick D, McCoy E, McGregor D, Mortelmans K, Rosenkranz HS, Simmon VF (1985) Reproducibility of microbial mutagenicity assays: II. Testing of carcinogens and noncarcinogens in *Salmonella typhimurium* and *Escherichia coli*. Environ. Mutagen. 7 (suppl. 5):1-248.

Gold LS, Wright C, Bernstein L, de Veciana M (1987) Reproducibility of results in "near-replicate" carcinogenicity bioassays. J. Nat. Cancer Inst. 78:1149-1158.

Gross ST (1986) The kappa coefficient of agreement for multiple observers when the number of subjects is small. Biometrics 42:883-893.

Haworth S, Lawtor T, Mortelmans K, Speck W, Zeiger E (1983) Salmonella mutagenicity results for 250 chemicals. Environ. Mutagen. 5 (suppl. 1):3-142.

Kupper LL, Hafner KB (1989) On assessing interrater agreement for multiple attribute response. Biometrics 45:957-967.

Mortelmans K, Haworth S, Lawlor T, Speck W, Tainer B, Zeiger E (1986) Salmonella mutagenicity tests: II. Results from the testing of 270 chemicals. Environ. Mutagen. 8 (suppl. 7):1-119.

Zeiger E, Anderson B, Haworth S, Lawlor T (1988) Salmonella mutagenicity tests: IV. Results from the testing of 300 chemicals. Environ. Mutagen. 11 (suppl. 12):1-158.

Zeiger E, Anderson B, Haworth S, Lawlor T, Mortelmans K, Speck W (1987) Salmonella mutagenicity tests: III. Results from the testing of 255 chemicals. Environ. Mutagen. 9 (suppl. 9):1-109.

Table 1. Qualitative reproducibility of *Salmonella* mutagenicity

Chemical	+	+W	-	?	Chemical	+	+W	-	?
Acetaldehyde	0	0	2	0	Acetonitrile	0	0	2	0
Acrylamide	0	1	1	0	AF-2	10	0	0	0
Aflatoxin (N1D-82107)	2	0	0	0	Allyl acrylate	0	0	2	0
Allyl isothiocyanate	0	1	1	0	9-Aminoacridine HCl H_2O	3	0	0	0
2-Aminoanthracene	7	0	0	0	2-Aminobiphenyl	11	0	1	0
4-Aminobiphenyl	3	0	0	0	2-Amino-6-MBT	2	0	0	0
2-Amino-6-NBT	2	0	0	0	2-Amino-4-nitrophenol	2	0	0	0
o-Aminophenol	2	1	0	0	p-Aminophenol	0	0	3	0
n-Amyl nitrite	4	2	0	0	m-Anisidine	1	1	1	0
o-Anisidine	2	0	0	1	p-Anisidine	2	0	1	0
Anthracene	0	2	0	0	L-Ascorbic acid	0	1	1	0
Azobenzene	2	0	0	0	Benzamide	0	0	2	0
Benzidine	5	0	0	0	Benzoin	0	1	2	0
Benzonitrile	0	0	2	0	Benzo(a)pyrene	2	0	0	0
Benzo(f)quinoline	1	0	0	1	Benzyl chloride	0	2	0	0
o-Benzyl-p-chlorophenol	0	0	2	0	Benzyl salicylate	0	0	2	0
Biphenyl	0	0	2	0	Bis(2-chloroethyl)ether	0	1	0	1
BCME	4	1	0	0	Bisphenol A	0	0	3	0
Boric acid	0	0	1	1	Bromochloromethane	2	0	0	0
α-Bromo-α-EBU	0	0	2	0	Bromoform	0	0	1	2
Butyl benzyl phthalate	0	0	2	0	Butyraldehyde	0	0	2	0
Calcium chromate, anhydrous	4	1	0	1	Calcium cyanamide	0	1	0	1
Carbon disulfide	0	0	2	0	Carbon tetrachloride	0	0	2	0
Carminic acid	0	3	0	0	Catechol (1,2-Benzenediol)	0	0	2	0
m-Chloroaniline	0	0	2	0	o-Chloroaniline	0	0	2	0
p-Chloroaniline	1	1	1	0	o-Chlorobenzalmalononitrile	0	0	0	2
Chlorobenzene	0	0	2	0	Chlorobenzilate	0	0	2	0
2-Chloroethanol	2	0	0	0	2-CETA Cl	0	0	2	0
3-Chloro-2-methylpropene	0	1	2	0	2-Chloronitrobenzene	2	1	0	0
4-Chloronitrobenzene	2	0	0	0	Chloropicrin	2	0	0	0
1-Chloro-2-propanol	3	0	0	0	3-Chloro-p-toluidine	0	1	1	0

Table 1. Qualitative reproducibility of *Salmonella* mutagenicity (cont'd)

Chemical	+	+W	-	?	Chemical	+	+W	-	?
Chlorotrianisene	0	0	2	0	Chlorotrimethyl silane	0	1	1	0
Choline chloride	0	0	3	0	Citral diethyl acetal	1	0	1	0
Cyclohexanone	0	0	2	0	Cyclophosphamide monohydrate	2	0	0	0
2,4-D	0	0	2	0	D&C yellow 11	0	1	0	1
n-Decane	0	0	1	1	Diallyl phthalate	0	0	2	0
1,6-Diaminohexane	0	0	2	0	Dibromoacetonitrile	0	3	0	1
Dibromomannitol	2	0	0	0	N,N'-Di-sec-butyl-p-PD	0	0	2	0
cis-1,2-Dichloroethylene	0	0	2	0	Dichloromethotrexate	0	1	2	0
2,3-Dichloronitrobenzene	0	2	0	0	1,2-Dichloropropane	0	2	0	0
5-Diethylamino-2-NP HCl	0	0	2	0	DEHA	0	0	2	0
DEHP	0	0	5	0	Diethyl phthalate	0	0	2	0
Di(n-hexyl)phthalate	0	0	2	0	Diisodecyl phthalate	0	0	2	0
Dimenhydrinate	1	0	0	1	Dimethoate (Cygon)	2	0	0	0
3,3'-Dimethoxybenzidine	3	0	0	0	Dimethylamine	0	0	2	0
Dimethylcarbamoyl chloride	5	0	0	0	Dimethyl cyanamide	0	0	2	0
Dimethylethanolamine	0	0	1	1	Dimethyl hydrogenphosphite	0	1	0	1
2,6-Dimethyl morpholine	1	0	1	0	DMOHE urea	1	0	1	0
2,4-Dimethyl phenol	0	1	1	0	Dimethylsulfoxide (DMSO)	0	0	2	0
1,3-Dioxane	0	1	0	1	1,4-Dioxane	0	0	2	0
Diphenylhydantoin	0	0	2	0	Direct black 38; C.I. 30235	2	0	0	0
Direct blue 6; C.I. 22610	0	0	2	0	Direct brown 95; C.I. 30145	0	1	1	0
2,2'-Dithiobisbenzothiazole	2	0	0	0	Divinylbenzene	0	0	2	0
9,10-EOD acid, 2-EH ester	0	0	1	1	1,2-Epoxypropane	2	0	0	0
1,2-Epoxy-3,3,3-TCP	2	0	0	0	Ethyl acrylate (inhibited)	0	1	2	0
Ethylenediamine	4	2	0	1	Ethylene thiourea	0	1	1	0
2-Ethylhexyl acrylate	0	0	2	0	Ethylidene norbornene	0	0	2	0
Ethyl tellurac	0	0	2	0	Fenthion	0	1	1	0
Ferrocene	0	0	1	1	Formaldehyde	5	2	0	0
Formamide	0	0	2	0	Formanilide	0	0	2	0
Furfural	0	0	1	1	Gallic acid	0	0	1	1
Glutaric dialdehyde	0	1	0	1	Glycerol	0	0	2	1
Glycidol	2	0	0	0	Glycine	0	0	2	0
Hexabromobenzene	0	0	2	0	Hexabromobiphenyl	0	0	2	0
Hexachloroethane	0	0	2	0	Hexanamide	0	0	1	1
1,6-Hexanediol diacrylate	0	0	2	0	p-Hexylresorcinol	0	0	2	0
Hydroquinone monometh. ether	0	0	2	0	2-Hydroxybenzamide	0	0	2	0
N-Hydroxybenzamide	2	0	0	0	2-Hydroxy-4-MOBP	0	1	1	0
3-Hydroxypropanenitrile	0	0	2	0	FD&C Blue 2; C.I. 73015	1	1	0	0
Iodoform	2	0	0	0	Isatin-5-sulfonic acid	1	1	0	0
Isobutyl nitrite	3	0	0	0	Isoproterenol hydrochloride	0	1	1	0
D-Limonene dimercaptan	0	0	3	0	Manganese sulfate, monohydr.	0	0	2	0
Mannitol	0	0	4	0	2-Mercaptobenzothiazole	0	0	1	1
Methacrylonitrile	0	0	2	0	Methdilazine HCl	0	0	2	0
Methoxychlor	0	0	2	0	2-Methoxyethyl acetate	0	1	0	1
o-Methoxyphenol	0	0	3	0	Methyl acrylate	0	0	2	0
N-Methyl-p-AP sulfate	1	1	0	0	2-Methyl-2-butenenitrile	0	0	2	0
2-Methyl-3-butenenitrile	0	1	1	0	3-Methylcholanthrene	3	0	0	0
2'-Methyl-4-DMAA	0	0	0	2	MOCA	8	1	0	1
Methyl isocyanate	0	0	2	0	Methyl methacrylate	0	0	2	0
Methylphenidate HCl	0	0	2	0	N-Methyl-2-pyrrolidone	0	0	2	0
4-(2-Naphthylamino)phenol	0	0	1	1	Ninhydrin	0	0	1	1
p-Nitroaniline	2	0	0	0	o-Nitroanisole	2	0	0	0
4-Nitroanthranilic acid	2	0	0	0	Nitrobenzene	0	0	2	0
m-Nitrobenzoic acid	2	0	0	0	1-Nitrobutane	0	0	2	0
2-Nitroethanol	1	0	0	1	Nitrofurantoin	7	0	0	0
o-Nitrophenethyl alcohol	2	0	1	0	o-Nitrophenol	0	0	2	0
4-Nitro-o-phenylenediamine	3	0	0	0	1-Nitropropane	0	0	2	0
2-Nitropropane	4	0	0	0	N-Nitrosodimethylamine	4	0	0	0
N-Nitrosopiperidine	10	0	0	0	o-Nitrotoluene	0	0	2	0

Table 1. Qualitative reproducibility of *Salmonella* mutagenicity (cont'd)

Chemical	+	+W	-	?	Chemical	+	+W	-	?
NPDPP, mixed isomers	0	0	2	1	2-Octyl-3-isothiazolone	0	0	2	0
n-Octyl methacrylate	0	0	1	1	Parathion	0	1	1	0
2-Pentenenitrile	0	0	1	1	Pheniramine maleate	0	0	2	0
Phenol	0	0	2	0	Phenolphthalein	0	0	2	0
Phenylacetonitrile	0	0	2	0	Phenyl mercuric acetate	0	0	1	1
o-Phenylphenol	0	1	1	0	Phenyl salicylate	0	0	1	1
Phthalic anhydride	0	0	2	0	Pigment violet 1	0	0	2	0
Potassium chloride	0	0	5	0	Prednisone	2	0	0	0
Promethazine HCl	0	0	2	0	Propantheline bromide	0	0	2	0
beta-Propiolactone	5	0	0	0	Propionitrile	0	0	2	0
1,2-Propylene glycol	0	0	2	0	Quinidine	0	0	2	0
p-Quinone	0	0	2	0	Resorcine blue	0	0	2	0
Ricinoleic acid, Na salt	0	0	2	0	Sodium chloride	0	0	2	0
Sodium phosphate, dibasic	0	0	5	0	Streptomycin sulfate (2:3)	0	2	1	0
Succinic anhydride	0	0	2	0	Succinonitrile	0	0	2	0
Sulfamethizole	0	0	2	0	5-Sulfoanthranilic acid	0	0	1	1
2,4,5-T	0	0	2	0	2,3,5,6-TCNB	0	2	0	0
Tetrachlorophthalic anhydr.	0	0	2	0	Tetraethyl lead	0	0	2	0
Tetrahydrofuran	0	0	2	0	N,N,N',N'-Tetramethyl-p-PD	2	0	0	0
2,2'-Thiobis(4,6-DCP)	0	0	1	1	Thiocarbanilide	0	0	1	1
Thiophene	0	0	2	0	o-Toluidine HCl	1	0	1	0
Triamterene	0	0	2	0	Tributyl borate	0	0	2	0
Tributyl phosphate	0	0	2	0	Trichloroacetonitrile	0	2	0	0
2,4,6-Trichloroaniline	0	1	1	0	1,1,1-Trichloroethane	0	0	4	0
1,1,2-Trichloroethane	0	0	2	0	1,2,3-Trichloropropane	2	0	0	0
Tricresyl phosphate	0	0	2	0	Triphenylamine	0	0	2	0
Tris(2-CE)phosphite	0	1	0	1	Tris(1,3-DC-2-P)phosphate	8	0	0	0
Vat blue 1; C.I. 73000	1	0	0	1	Water	0	1	2	0
Hamamelis water	1	0	3	0	2,6-Xylidine	0	2	1	0
Zinc pyrithione	0	0	2	0					

Abbreviations

2-Amino-6-MBT:	2-Amino-6-methoxybenzothiazole
2-Amino-6-NBT:	2-Amino-6-nitrobenzothiazole
AF-2:	2-(2-Furyl)-3-(5-nitro-2-furyl)acrylamide
BCME	Bis(2-chloro-1-methylethyl)ether
α-Bromo-α-EBU:	alpha-Bromo-alpha-ethylbutyrylurea
2-CETA Cl:	2-Chloroethyl trimethyl ammonium Cl
2,4-D:	2,4-Dichlorophenoxyacetic acid
N,N'-Di-sec-butyl-p-PD:	N,N'-Di-sec-butyl-p-phenylenediamine
5-Diethylamino-2-NP HCl:	5-Diethylamino-2-nitrosophenol HCl
DEHA:	Di(2-ethylhexyl)adipate
DEHAP:	Di(2-ethylhexyl)phthalate
DMOHE:	Dimethyloldihydroxyethylene urea
9,10-EOD acid, 2-EH ester:	9,10-Epoxyoctadecanoic acid, 2-ethylhexyl ester
1,2-Epoxy-3,3,3-TCP:	1,2-Epoxy-3,3,3-trichloropropane
2-Hydroxy-4-MOBP:	2-Hydroxy-4-methoxybenzophenone
N-Methyl-p-AP sulfate:	N-Methyl-p-aminophenol sulfate
2'-Methyl-4-DMAA:	2'-Methyl-4-dimethylaminoazobenzene
MOCA:	4,4'-Methylene-bis-2-chloroaniline
NPDPP:	Nonylphenyl diphenyl phosphate
2,4,5-T:	2,4,5-Trichlorophenoxyacetic acid
2,3,5,6-TCNB:	2,3,5,6-Tetrachloronitrobenzene
N,N,N',N'-Tetramethyl-p-PD:	N,N,N',N'-Tetramethyl-p-phenylenediamine
2,2'-Thiobis(4,6-DCP):	2,2'-Thiobis(4,6-dichlorophenol)
Tris(2-CE)phosphite:	Tris(2-chloroethyl)phosphite
Tris(1,3-DC-2-P)phosphate:	Tris(1,3-dichloro-2-propyl)phosphate

TABULAR OVERVIEW OF STATISTICAL METHODS PROPOSED FOR THE ANALYSIS OF AMES *SALMONELLA* ASSAY DATA

Joachim Vollmar and Lutz Edler

Boehringer Mannheim GmbH, D-6800 Mannheim, Germany

National Institute of Environmental Health Sciences, Research Triangle Park, NC 27709, USA

Introduction to the Table

The AMES *Salmonella*/Microsome assay has challenged considerable biometrical efforts for data analysis since its introduction to mutagenicity testing in 1975. Approaches proposed by various authors range from straightforward applications of classical linear models to more sophisticated statistical methods such as those of generalized linear models. The assay motivated the use of stochastic branching process theory for constructing the model equations to analyze mutagenicity data, and it is considered as an important example of the analysis of overdispersed count data. Non-parametric methods have also been applied with success.

Table 1 gives an overview of tests and estimation procedures proposed for the Ames mutagenicity assay. It updates an earlier compilation (Vollmar, 1985) and an attempt was made to include most of the statistical techniques suggested for the analysis of the revertant count data from Ames assay. Since the literature on this assay is huge and still increasing, we cannot be sure of having considered all existing statistical methodology for this subject, nevertheless, we are convinced that we present those which are of highest statistical importance. Yet, ongoing statistical research on the analysis of Ames-type data may still provide improved methods in the future. We should mention here also the review of statistical methods for microbial test sytems by Mahon et al (1989) mainly devoted to the Ames assay.

Hundreds of short-term tests have been introduced since the introduction of the Ames *Salmonella* assay (Waters et al, 1987). An overview of appropriate statistical methods for some of them has been given recently in the monograph edited by Kirkland (1989). It is interesting to see research for adequate statistical methods for other mutagenicity assays following to some extent the lines of the Ames assay. Therefore, our list also provides guidelines for the application or invention of biometric methods for other short-term tests.

The table below has been organized into four parts. The first section (A) exhibits the earliest methods; methods which were mostly qualitative and designed for testing differences between control and dose groups. More efficient methods are listed in section (B) for the assay's investigation by non-parametric methods and in section (C) for its analysis by parametric regression methods applied to various models of the revertant count data. Methods for the joint action of at least two mutagens are deferred to section (D). For reasons of clarity we characterized the methods by a very few key words only, except in (C), where crude model equations are given. There, y denotes the number of revertants per plate, d the dose or concentration, and a,b,c,p and γ respective regression parameters. Distributional assumptions are listed for parametric models. For more detail we recommend the study of the the original publication.

Acknowledgements

Thanks are due Drs Walter Piegorsch, Christopher Portier and Paige Williams for their helpful remarks in preparing the table.

Table 1: Statistical Methods for Ames *Salmonella* Assay

A) Qualitative Analysis without Dose-Response Model

Method	*Distribution*	*Authors*
Multiple t-tests in many-to-one design	Normal	Ehrenberg, 1977
Tolerance interval for spontaneous counts	Normal	Andrews et al, 1978;
ANOVA[1], transformation of counts		Weinstein&Lewinson,1978;
Comparison of frequencies	Binomial/Poisson	Katz, 1979;
Wilcoxon rank sum test	-	Vollmar, 1981;
Two-sample Kolmogorov-Smirnov test	-	Mitchell, 1982;
Nemenyi / Maximum test	-	Schumacher, 1985;

B) Qualitative Analysis with Monotone Dose-Response Model

Method	*Authors*
Jonckheere test	Vollmar, 1981;
Chacko-Shorak test	Vollmar, 1981 Schumacher, 1985;
Isotonic regression	Collings et al, 1981;
Modified Page test	Wahrendorf et al , 1984;
Adaptive test procedure for the Wilcoxon rank sum and Jonckheere test	Simpson&Margolin, 1986 Schmoor&Schumacher, 1988 Simpson&Margolin, 1990;

C) Quantiative Analysis with Dose-Response Model

Model[6]	*Method*	*Distribution*	*Authors*
$y = a + bd$	Linear regression	Normal	Benedict et al, 1977;
	Adaptive procedure with LR^2 test	Neg. Binomial	Bernstein et al, 1982;
	Stepwise linear regression	Normal	Venitt, 1982;
	Linear regression after eliminating toxic doses	Normal	Moore&Felton, 1983;
	Modified quasi-likelihood	Mean-variance relationship	Schmoor& Schumacher, 1988;
$y = a + blnd$ [7]	Linear regression	Normal	Andrews et al, 1978;
$ln(y - y_0) = a + blnd$ [7]	Linear regression	Normal	Brusick, 1977;
$lny = a + bln(d+1)$	Linear regression after eliminating outliers and toxic doses	Normal	Chu et al, 1981;
$(y+1)^p = a + d$	Linear regression after Box-Cox transformation	Normal	Snee&Irr, 1984;
$y = (a + bd) \times exp(-\gamma d)$	Weighted least squares variance heterogeneity	Normal	Myers et al, 1981;

$y = (a+bd^c) \times exp(-\gamma d)$ $y = (a+bd^c)$	MLE[3] and iterative modified Gauss-Newton method, LR[2] for goodness of fit,	Poisson	Stead et al, 1981
	weighted LS[4], confidence bounds, SAS program	Normal	Alvord et al, 1990;
$y = a+b(1-e^{-cd}) \times e^{-\gamma d}$	Branching model, MLE[3]	Neg. Binomial	Margolin et al, 1981;
$lny = a+bln(d+c) - \gamma d$	GLM[5], iterative procedure quasi-likelihood methods	Extra Poisson exponential family	Breslow, 1984, 1990 Breslow&Kaldor, 1986;

D) Quantitative Analysis of Joint Action of Two Mutagens

Method	*Authors*
Simple independent action model $lnQ_{AB} = lnQ_A + lnQ_B - lnQ_0$	Piegorsch&Margolin, 1989;
Simple similar action model $-ln\left(\frac{\pi_{ab}}{1-\pi_{ab}}\right) = \mu + \beta_1 d_a + \beta_2 d_b$	Chen et al, 1989.

Legend

[1]ANOVA analysis of variance
[2]LR likelihood ratio test
[3]MLE maximum likelihood estimation
[4]LS least squares estimation
[5]GLM generalized linear model

[6] y = number of revertants per plate
y_0 = y-value at dose 0
d = dose/concentration

[7] for $d > 0$ only

References

Alvord WG, Driver JH, Claxton L, Creason JP (1990) Methods for comparing *Salmonella* mutagenicity data sets using nonlinear models. Mutat. Res. 240: 177-194

Andrews AW, Thibault LH, Ljinski W (1978) The relationship between carcinogenicity and mutagenicity of some polynuclear hydrocarbons. Mutat. Res. 51: 319-326

Benedict WF, Baker MS, Haroun L, Choi W, Ames BN (1977) Mutagenicity of cancer chemotherapeutic agents in the *Salmonella*/microsome test. Cancer Res. 37: 2209-2213

Bernstein L, Kaldor J, McCann J, Pike MC (1982) An empirical approach to the statistical analysis of mutagenesis data from the Salmonella test. Mutat. Res. 97: 267-281

Breslow NE (1984) Extra-Poisson variation in log-linear models. Appl. Statist. 33: 38-44

Breslow NE (1990) Tests of hypotheses in overdispersed Poisson regression and other quasi-likelihood models. J. Amer Statist. Assoc. 85: 565-571

Breslow NE, Kaldor J (1986) Statistical analysis of data from in-vitro assays of mutagenesis. In Montesano R, Bartsch H, Vainio H, Wilbourn J, Yamasaki H (eds) Long-term and Short-term assays for Carcinogens: A Critical Appraisal. IARC Sci Publications, IARC Lyon, 457-481

Brusick DJ (1977) In vitro mutagenesis assays as predictors of chemical carcinogenesis in mammals. Clin. Toxicol. 10: 79-109

Chen JJ, Heflich RH, Hass BS (1989) A response-additive model for analyzing mixtures of two chemicals in the *Salmonella* reversion assay. Biom. J. 31: 495-503

Chu KC, Patel KM, Lin AH, Tarone RE, Lin MS, Dunkel VC (1981) Evaluating statistical analyses and reproducibility of microbial mutagenicity assays. Mutat. Res. 85: 119-132

Collings BJ, Margolin BH, Oehlert GW (1981) Analyses of binomial data with application to the fluctuation test for mutagenicity. Biometrics 37: 775-794

Ehrenberg L (1977) Aspects of statistical inference in testing for genetic toxicity. In: Kilbey BJ, Legator M, Ramel C (eds) Handbook of Mutagenicity Test Procedures. Elsevier, Amsterdam, 419-459

Katz AJ (1979) Design and analysis of experiments on mutagenicity II. Assays involving micro-organisms. Mutat. Res. 64, 61-77

Kirkland DJ (1989) Statistical Evaluation of Mutagenicity Test Data. Cambridge University Press, Cambridge

Mahon GAT, Green MHL, Middleton B, Mitchell I de G, Robinson WD, Tweats DJ (1989) Analysis of data from microbial colony assays. In: Kirkland DJ (ed) Statistical Evaluation of Mutagenicity Test Data. Cambridge University Press, Cambridge, 26-65

Margolin BH, Kaplan N, Zeiger E (1981) Statistical analysis of the Ames *Salmonella*/microsome test. Proc. Natl. Acad. Sci. 78: 3779-3783

Mitchell I de G (1982) Establishment of stochastic significance in Ames tests and its relevance to genetical significance. Mutat. Res. 104: 25-28

Moore D, Felton JS (1983) A microcomputer program for analyzing Ames test data. Mutat. Res. 119: 95-102

Myers LE, Sexton NH, Southerland LI, Wolff TJ (1981) Regression analysis of Ames test data. Environ. Mutagen. 3: 575-586

Piegorsch WW, Margolin (1989) Quantitative methods for assessing a synergistic or potentiated genotoxic response. Mutat. Res. 216: 1-8

Schmoor C, Schumacher M (1988) Adaptive statistical procedures for the analysis of mutagenicity data. Institute of Medical Biometry and Informatics, University of Freiburg. December 1988.

Schumacher M (1985) Statistische Analyse des Ames Tests. Universitaet Dortmund, Arbeitsberichte der Abt. Statistik No. 18

Simpson DG, Margolin BH (1986) Recursive nonparametric testing for dose-response relationships subject to downturns at high doses. Biometrika 73: 589-596

Simpson DG, Margolin BH (1990) Nonparametric testing for dose-response curves subject to downturns: asymptotic power considerations. Ann. Statist. 18: 373-390

Snee RD, Irr JD (1984) A procedure for the statistical evaluation of Ames *Salmonella* assay results: comparison of results among four laboratories. Mutat. Res. 128: 115-125

Stead AG, Hasselblad V, Creason JP, Claxton L (1981) Modeling the Ames test. Mutat. Res. 85: 13-27.

Venitt S (1982) UKEMS collaborative genotoxicity trial - bacterial mutation tests of 4-chloromethylbiphenyl, 4-hydroxymethylbiphenyl and benzyl chloride; analysis of data from 17 laboratories. Mutat. Res. 100: 91-109

Vollmar J (1981): Statistical problems in the Ames test. In: Kappas A (ed) Progress in Mutation Research . Elsevier, Amsterdam, 179-186

Vollmar J (1985) Nichtparametrische Trendtests in der Mutagenitaetspruefung. Kolloquium "Statistische Methoden in der experimentellen Forschung", TU Berlin

Wahrendorf J, Mahon GAT, Schumacher M (1985) A nonparametric approach to the statistical analysis of mutagenicity data. Mutat. Res. 147: 5-13

Waters MD, Stack HF, Brady AL, Lohmann, PHM, Haroun L, Vainio H (1987) Activity profiles for genetic and related tests. In: IARC Monographs on the Evaluation of Carcinogenic Risks to Humans. Genetic and Related Effects: An Updating of Selected IARC Monographs from Volumes 1-42. Supplement 6. IARC Lyon, Appendix 1, 687-696

Weinstein D, Lewinson TM (1978) A statistical treatment of the Ames mutagenicity assay. Mutat. Res. 51: 433-434

ANALYSES OF LONGTERM CARCINOGENICITY STUDIES

Jörg Kaufmann

Schering AG, HD Biometrie, Müllerstr. 170-175, D-1000 Berlin 65

The statistical analysis of tumor and survival data is an essential component of the evaluation of carcinogenicity. Care must be taken, in assessing carcinogenic potential, not to place total reliance on the finding of statistically significant results.

The basic premise of cognition through planned experiments is that the hypotheses to be tested are set before beginning the study. Nevertheless, there is no reason why an ex post facto explorative data analysis cannot be performed.

Time adjusted analyses of crude proportions are necessary to eliminate the bias associated with the differential mortality. A time adjusted analysis is more appropriate and possibly more powerful. Several methods may be suggested.

The results of the "Peto statistic", a combined analysis of lethal and nonlethal tumors, are very similar to the results of the life table adjusted analysis in tumor bearing animals.

Introduction

The purpose of a chemical carcinogen bioassay is to determine whether the chemical to be tested has a carcinogenic potential. The role of the biometrician in the decision process is two-fold: to participate in the planning of experiments and to analyse the carcinogenicity data.

The basic data obtained from each animal are the time of death, the cause of death (in so far as the causes can be determined) and the histopathological diagnoses of the examined organs. The statistical methods described are not new, though they are not yet widely correctly applied by experimentalists.

Mice and rats are the most common subjects of tumorgenicity studies, but dogs and monkeys are also used for specific substances, e.g., steroid hormones.

The test animals are observed for a major portion of their lifespan, for example

mice	-	78 to 104 weeks
rats	-	104 weeks
(dogs	-	7 years)
(monkeys	-	10 years)

The term "experimental unit" refers to the smallest unit of experimental material which is randomized identically. In the completely randomized design, the individual animal is the experimental unit.

All animals that die during the study are subjected to necropsy. At termination, all surviving animals are killed and subjected to necropsy.

The experiment is terminated according to a predetermined stopping rule, e.g., after a fixed period of time (see above), or when mortality in the control or lowest-dose group exceeds a specified limit such as 60%.

Dose selection

In a typical longterm carcinogenicity experiment, a pool of animals is divided by randomization into several groups. One group serves as a concurrent control group, while the remaining groups are exposed to various dose levels of the test substance.

Dose selection is one of the most controversial and important elements for a chronic bioassay. In studies screening for potential carcinogens, the biological ideal would be to test only dose levels comparable to those to which humans are exposed. However, this is not practical for economic reasons. A substance that causes the rate of some cancers to increase from 1% to 2% might not be detected as a carcinogen even in a relatively large animal experiment.

Test of Hypotheses

Carcinogenic treatments usually affect a few types of tumor strongly and the remaining types hardly at all. For this reason it is usually advisable to carry out separate statistical analyses for each tumor type that occurs. But the basic premise of cognition through planned experiments is that the hypotheses are set before the study is begun. An additional implicit assumption is that an acceptable Type I error rate is chosen.

The false-positive and false-negative rates are of great importance in any screening procedure. In most animal carcinogenesis experiments, it is not possible to predict a priori potential target organs in which carcinogenic effects are likely to occur. Thus, although the effect of a carcinogenic agent is expected to be concentrated in one or a few target organs, all organs which are examined histopathologically must be evaluated for evidence of carcinogenesis.

Thus the hypotheses are usually formulated for general statements, e.g., for total number of tumor bearing animals or for the total number of animals with a malignant tumor, irrespective of site. The interpretation of a significant or non significant result is the general: "The substance is tumorigenic or not tumorigenic".

Of course, there is no reason why an ex post facto explorative data analysis cannot be performed. In any event, the results of such an analysis are to be viewed as suggestions for hypotheses for new studies or as suggestions for the existence of events. In no case such results are to be viewed as confirmatory.

Biometrical aspects

There is a number of situations in which the use of models based on time-to-tumor information has advantages. Overall proportions can be misleading, however, when survival distributions are different across treatment groups in an experiment. Suppose we can classify deaths as "early deaths" or "late deaths" as in the following 2 x 2 tables.

	"Early deaths"			"Late deaths"			Total	
	Control	Treated		Control	Treated		Control	Treated
Tumor	0	0	T	10	20	T	10	20
			+			=		
No Tumor	30	10		10	20	NT	40	30

Note that for both treated and control, there are no tumors observed for early deaths and the tumor rate is 50% among animals classified as dying late in the study. When summarized in a single 2 x 2 table, tumor rates are 20% in controls and 40% in the treated group, but there is really a difference in survival and not in tumor rates.

The above situation is an example where survival distributions are different across treatment groups, so that overall proportions can be misleading.

Time-to-tumor models may allow graphical presentation of the observed and fitted time curves for tumor onset in treatment. Control groups can be used to indicate whether there might be any interaction between the effect of treatment and time.

In the past, time-to-tumor models have mainly been applied to visible tumors. However, in recent years a number of attempts have been made to consider the more general situation where tumors may also be fatal or incidental.

A schematic presentation of the tumor-death model is provided in Fig. 1, where the possible states in which an animal can be are given as boxes along with possible transitions (arrows) in the proposed model.

It is assumed that an animal is in the normal state, N, at the beginning of the experiment, from which it can transfer either to the tumor state, T, or to the state D_{CR}, representing death from a competing risk, or to the state TS, representing survival until the end of the study.

An animal in state T can either die because of the tumor and so transfer to the state D_T, or it can die of a competing risk and so move to state D_{CR}. It is assumed that the tumor is an irreversible disease, and therefore the model does not allow a transfer from state T to state N. At the end of the experiment, all surviving animals are killed and so transfer to the state TS.

The assumption that a transition is made from a normal state to a state where the tumor is detectable is simplistic. Even in the model proposed, the information on cause of death, required to distinguish between D_T and D_{CR} when a tumor is present, is often difficult if not impossible to obtain.

The goal of most carcinogenicity studies is to compare tumor rates in control animals to tumor rates in treated animals. The most appropriate basis for this comparison is the tumor incidence rate. The tumor rate is the frequency of tumor bearing animals in the corresponding treatment group. Another important rate used in analyzing is the mortality rate in the presence of tumor.

The absence or presence of a tumor and the rate of death in tumor-bearing animals are functions of both the tumor incidence rate and the mortality rate.

The mortality rate can be separated into two types: The mortality rate in tumor-free animals and the mortality rate in tumor-bearing animals (Fig. 2).

Time adjusted analyses of crude proportion

Time adjusted analyses are necessary to eliminate the bias associated with the differential mortality and thus to ensure the validity of statistical tests.

Several methods have been suggested for taking the time variable into account. One starts with a simple procedure; later a more sophisticated procedure in the life table or survival adjusted analysis will be presented.

The asymptotic relative efficiency (ARE) between test on proportions (TP) and log rank test (LRT) is ARE(TP/LRT) ~ 98 % for a tumor rate of 0.4, that is both tests are equally sufficient for practical use (L. Hothorn (1989), J. Cuzik (1982)).

Adjusted proportions with tumors are formed, having the same numerators and the suitable diminished denominators. There are three alternative ways of choosing the denominator (Gart et.al. (1986)).

1) The number of animals initially tested in each group.

2) The number initially tested, less the number of animals which were not subjected to necrospy or for which the organ site in question was not submitted to or yielded tissue slides unsuitable for pathological examination. Thus, for instance, those animals whose lungs were not available for pathological examination would be excluded from the denominators (in the analyses of lung tumors) but if their livers were examined, they would be included in the denominators of the analysis of liver tumors. In such cases, the denominators may vary from tumor site to tumor site within the same experiment.

3) The initial number at risk, less those animals not subjected to necropsy or for which tissue slides for the organ in question are missing, and less, also those animals dying early.

Early death may be defined in at least two ways:

3a) Death before a pre-specified time on test, say half year. In this case no death with tumor is expected to occur during the first 6 months of the study. Of course, if a tumor is found before this time, one should use the next option.

3b) Death before the first tumor at a specific site is found in any of the groups being compared.

Alternatives (2) and (3) imply that the missing animals or those dying early are as likely to have had the tumor their full life time as those that survived to terminal sacrifice and underwent a necropsy.

A Fisher exact test may be used to compare separately the tumor incidence in each treated group with a control group. In addition to the individual pairwise comparisons with control, an overall comparison among all the groups may be done. This test may be done either as an exact generalization of the Fisher-test or as a trend test. This trend test determines whether the incidence of tumor rises or falls from control group through the group given low dose, and finally to the group given high dose.

Nonparametric analysis of survival curves

In carcinogenecity experiments we observe the time of death and an indicator of the presence or absence of the tumor. For each tumor type and site, a "survival curve without apparent tumor" can be calculated for each group by means of Kaplan-Meier methods. In this calculation the weeks of death of animals dying with tumor are entered as a response and the weeks of death of animals dying without tumors are entered as censored observations. The terminal kill data may be entered in the same way as the data for those animals dying naturally. Suppose that observations of the experimental endpoint of interest (e.g., death with tumor) are made at H distinct times t_h, $h=1,...,H$. The data corresponding to each experimental endpoint may be summarized in H 2 x (I+1) contingency tables ($H \geq 1$), for a study with I dose group and one control group. (Table 1)

The X_{ih} denotes the number of events (death with tumor) observed in the ith group at t_h, and n_{ih} denotes the number of animals at risk in group i, for h=1,...,H.

Then, the Kaplan-Meier estimator of the survival function for group i is the step function defined as:

$$\hat{S}_i(t) = 1 \qquad \text{for } t \leq t_1$$

$$\hat{S}_i(t) = \prod_{h=1}^{H} \left(\frac{n_{ih} - x_{ih}}{n_{ih}}\right) \qquad \text{for } t > t_1$$

A plot of the (I+1) estimators $\hat{S}_i(t)$ from the beginning of the experiment until terminal sacrifice reveals any effects of exposure to the test compound on mortality. Estimates of the variance of $\hat{S}_i(t)$ and corresponding confidence interval can be calculated (Fig. 3)

Nonparametric test statistics

The most widely used statistic for testing survival differences is the generalized Savage statistic, often referred to as the log-rank statistic; the corresponding trend test statistic and departure from trend statistics were presented by Tarone. The modified Wilcoxon test of Breslow, the corresponding trend test statistic and departure from trend statistic are more sensitive than the generalized Savage statistics to differences in survival occurring early in an experiment, when a greater number of animals is at risk. (Table 2)

Comparison of the various adjusted tests of tumor incidence

The log rank or the modified Wilcoxon test on the one hand and the elimination of early death on the other may sometimes yield very different results. The life table tests detect the early observation of a tumor, whereas the other tests mainly detect differences in the relative tumor frequencies among groups.

When the observed time points indicate the onset of the tumor, the life table analyses test whether the treatment may induce not only more tumors, but also earlier tumors.

The higher dose may possibly induce more deaths earlier in a manner unrelated to the observed tumor, either by toxicity or by a lethal tumor at another site. Thus the tumors are observed earlier in the dead animals given the higher dose but may also be present in the same numbers of the animals that have not yet died and which received the lower dose.

Some writers have attempted to solve these difficulties by requiring that for each animal with tumor a decision should be made whether or not the tumor killed (lethal tumor) the animal. A slightly modified notion is to label certain tumors a priori as lethal and to use the life table tests on these tumors but to utilize the other time adjusted tests only on the nonlethal or "incidental" tumors.

Analysis of rapidly lethal tumors

Hoel and Walburg (1972) pointed out the importance of making a distinction between those tumors that are rapidly lethal and those that are nonlethal. Nonlethal occult tumors are discovered at necropsy, either after terminal sacrifice or after the animal has died because of illness unrelated to the presence of this kind of tumor.

We consider statistical methods that use the information on times to tumor, or more precisely, times to death because of tumor. The tumor when found at death is usually assumed to cause the death, even if the animal died accidentally or was sacrified because it was moribund.

For the terminal sacrifice the fatal/incidental distinction is not essential, since all animals that are killed at this terminal sacrifice were the only ones at risk of dying of a lethal tumor, and considering these tumors as either lethal or incidential will not alter the results.

The data are usually recorded in time units of days or weeks and are divided into sets labelled 'uncensored' or 'censored' for animals with and without tumors, respectively. The analysis requires specification of all time points at which tumors are found in any group, denoted by $t_1, \ldots, t_k$ (see above). The number of animals with tumor found at t_k in group i is denoted by y_{ik}. In general, the number at risk at t_k for group is m_{ik}. For experiments on lethal tumors, m_{ik} consists of all animals alive at the beginning of t_k, while for observable tumors m_{ik} excludes those living animals that already have a tumor.

The calculation of the Kaplan-Meier estimator of the survival function and the statistical tests for possible differences in these curves of survival are analogous to the formular given above if y_{ik} is substituted for x_{ik} and m_{ik} for n_{ik}.

Analysis for nonlethal occult tumors

Nonlethal occult tumors are discovered at necropsy, either after terminal sacrifice or after the animal has died prior to terminal sacrifice because of illness unrelated to the presence of the tumor. An assumption underlying the derivation of these tests is that, at least with regard to the presence or absence of a nonlethal tumor, death is a random sampling mechanism. This is an extremely strong assumption, that all tumors of a particular type observed in the carcinogenesis experiment under consideration are nonlethal.

Suppose the carcinogenesis experiment extends from time zero to time T, where T denotes the time at which the terminal sacrifice is scheduled. The interval (0, T) is subdivided into J-1 subintervals. Let the number of animals dying in group i during the jth subintervall be denoted by N_{ij} and the number of these animals in which a tumor is discovered at necropsy be denoted by Y_{ij}.

Test statistics can be computed using the log rank statistics after substituting J for K, j for k, Y_{ij} for X_{ik} and N_{ij} for n_{ik}. In the above analysis it was assumed that subdivisions were chosen a priori, without reference to the data on tumor prevalence.

Analysis of tumor data when contexts of observation are known

The analysis described earlier is valid if all tumors of a particular type are nonlethal and if all tumors of a particular type are rapidly lethal. The relationship between the presence of a tumor and death of most animals actually lies between these two extremes. If, however, one classifies deaths for each animal into one of the three categories

i) animal dies with tumor as cause of death,
ii) animal dies with tumor but from another cause or
iii) animals dies without tumor,

then the intermediate results obtained via the lethal and nonlethal analyses can be combined into an overall test incorporating cause of death.

Peto et al. (1980): suggest combining the (O-E) scores from the lethal analysis analysis with the (O-E) scores from the nonlethal or incidental analysis and also combining their variances.

As in the analysis of nonlethal tumors, the length of the experiment is subdivided into distinct time intervals. Within each time interval, the data on incidental tumors may be summarized in a table such as Table 1.

Form a vector $D_{NL} = (O-E)_{NL}$ of differences and compute the corresponding covariance matrix V_{NL}.

In the analysis of fatal tumors, animals in which the tumor is observed in the incidental context are treated exactly as all other animals not killed by the tumor. A vector $D_{LT} = (O-E)_{LT}$ of differences (lethal tumors) and the corresponding covariance matrix V_{LT} is computed.

The analysis of data on occult tumors using context of observation is based on the vector $D = D_{NL} + D_{LT}$ with covariance matrix $V = V_{NL} + V_{LT}$.

Test statistics for heterogenicity, trend and deviation from trend may be calculated as above (Gart et al. (1986)).

The results of the combined analysis of lethal and nonlethal tumors (Peto statistic) are very similar to the results of the life table adjusted analysis in tumor bearing animals. This is because the same number of tumor bearing animals is analyzed by both procedures. Furthermore, the computational procedures are also quite similar.

For some types of tumors there may be problems deciding whether or not they were fatal. Under these circumstances it may be advisable to class these tumors on a 4-point scale as suggested by Peto et al. (1980):

1 incidental
2 probably incidental
3 probably fatal
4 fatal .

Many alternative analyses can thereby be carried out for example, taking 1 (or 1 and 2) as incidental and 2, 3 and 4 (or 3 and 4) as fatal and then combining this into an overall test incorporating cause of death.

In the life table adjusted analysis the pathologist does not have the problem of classifying the tumor in the 4-point scale and the results are very similar.

References

Cuzik, J. (1982). The efficiency of the proportion test and log-rank test for consored survival data. Biometrics 38: 1033 - 1039.

Gart, J. J., Chu, K. C., Tarone, R. E. (1979) Statistical issues in the interpretation of chronic bioassay test for carcinogenicity Int. Cancer Inst., Vol. 62, 957 - 974

Gart, J. J., Krewski, D., Lee, P. N., Tarone, R. E., Wahrendort, J. (1986): Statistical methods in cancer research. Vol. III. The design and analysis of long-term animal experiment. International Agency for Research in Cancer.

Hoel, D. G., Walburg, H. E. (1972): Statistical analysis of survival experiments. Int. Cancer Inst. 49, 361 - 372

Hothorn, L. (1989). A simple statistical procedure for testing tumour rates in animal carcinogenicity experiments. Arch. Toxicol., Suppl. 13, 265 - 268

Kodell, R. L., Nelson, C. J. (1980) An illness-death model for the study of the Carcinogenic process using survival / sacrifice data. Biometrics, 36; 267 - 277

Passing, H., Dycka, J., Helmstädter, G., Kaufmann, J., Mau, J., Safer, A., Unkelbach, H. D., Vollmar, J., Wolf, Th. (1983): Zur statistischen Auswertung von Tumorigenitätsstudien. Biometrie in der chemisch-pharmazeutischen Industrie. Herausgeber: J. Vollmar, Gustav Fischer Verlag, 15 - 43.

Peto et al (1980): Guidelines for simple, sensitive significance test for carcinogenic effects in long-term animal experiments. Long-term and Short-term Screening Assays for Carcinogens: A Critical Appraisal. IARC Monographs, Supplement 2, 311 - 426.

Portier, C. J. (1988): Life table analysis of carcinogenicity experiments. Journal of the American College of Toxicology. Vol. 7, 575 - 582.

Selwyn, J. R. (1988): Preclinical safety development. Biopharmaceutical statistics for drug development. Edited: Karl E. Paece, Marcel Dekker, Inc. 246 - 258.

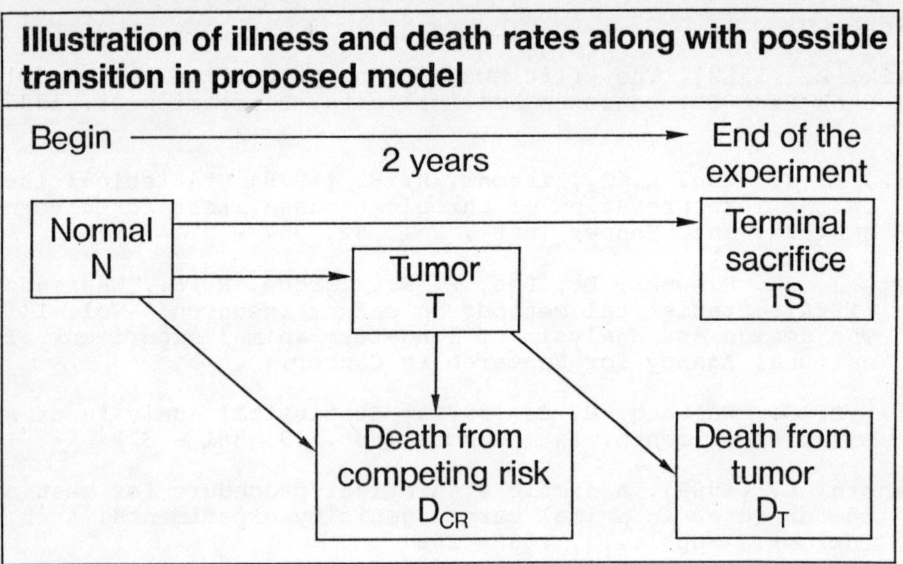

Figure 1: Illustration of illness and death rates along with possible transition in proposed model

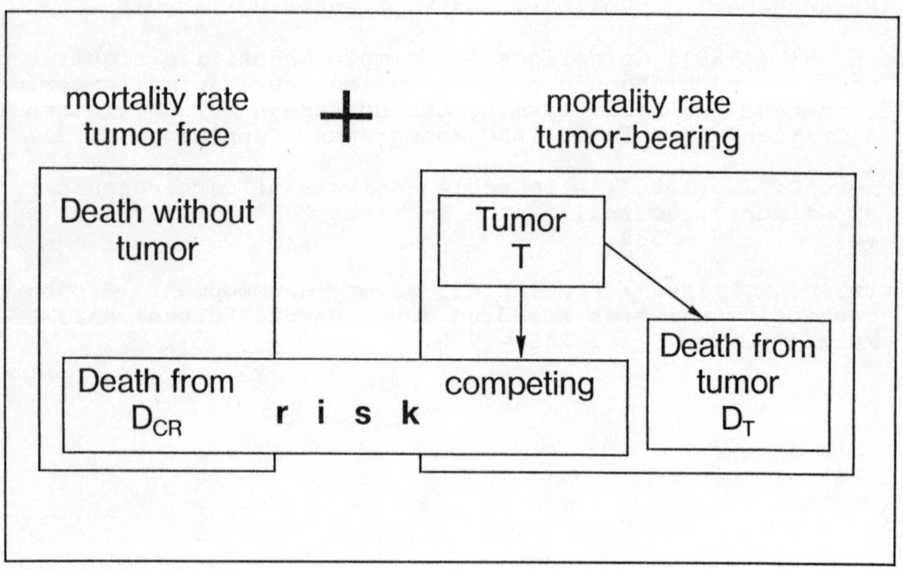

Figure 2: Mortality rate in tumor-free and tumor-bearing animals

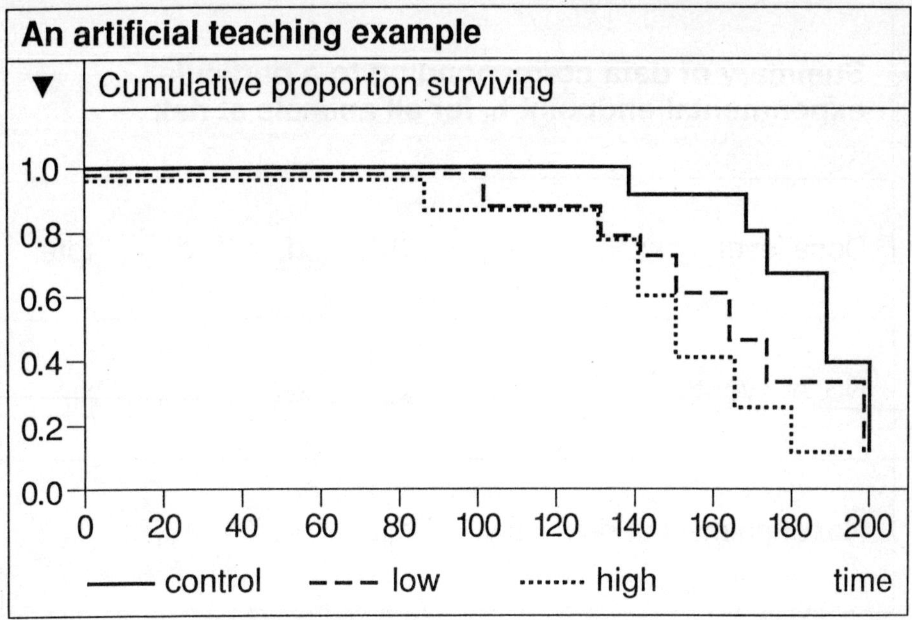

Figure 3: Kaplan-Meier estimator of the survival functions

Summary of data corresponding to a particular experimental endpoint t_h for all animals at risk					
Dose level	d_0	d_1	d_2	d_3	total
No. of events	x_{0h}	x_{1h}	x_{2h}	x_{3h}	x_h
No. of animals at risk	n_{0h}	n_{1h}	n_{2h}	n_{3h}	n_h

Table 1: Contingency table for an endpoint t_h.

Summary table teaching example							
	total	dead	1 dead	2 dead	3 dead	4 censored	proportion censored
control	15	2	2	0	2	9	0.6000
low	15	2	3	2	1	7	0.4667
high	15	2	1	2	3	7	0.4667
totals	45	6	6	4	6	23	

Test statistics			
	statistic	D.F.	P-value
generalized savage (Mantel-Cox)	4.557	2	0.1025
generalized Wilcoxon (Breslow)	5.695	2	0.0580
Test statisitcs for trend test			
Mantel-Cox (trend)	4.548	1	0.0330
Tarone-Ware (trend)	5.419	1	0.0199
Breslow (trend)	5.637	1	0.0176
Peto-Prentice (trend)	5.467	1	0.0194
coefficients for trend test are: -1.000 0.000 1.000			

Table 2: The most widely used statistic for testing survival differences

Mathematical models for the initiating and promotive action of carcinogens

Lars Ehrenberg and Gianpaolo Scalia-Tomba
Dept of Radiobiology and Dept of Mathematical Statistics
University of Stockholm, S-106 91 Stockholm

Introduction

Risk limitation has become an important issue to the public, administrators, and politicians in most societies. Systems for risk limitation have therefore been built up, particularly in industrialized countries. As indicated in O'Riordan's (1979) model, an important role in this process is played by the technology of risk assessment, which may be sub-divided into risk identification and risk estimation .

Risk estimation is required for decisions as to whether the magnitude of the harm caused by a factor is such that regulatory action is called for, and for risk-cost-benefit evaluations constituting the basis of the definition of acceptability and setting of permissible exposure limits on work premises and in the general environment.

Since, for cancer induced by chemicals and ionizing radiation, no threshold dose can be defined below which the risk is zero (Ehrenberg et al.,1983), the risk estimation is often concerned with very low exposure levels, down into the region where the associated risks are becoming acceptably low.

Considering the variations in sensitivity to carcinogenic processes, the individual cancer risk should be seen as the average probability of contracting, or dying from, the disease, the risk expectation ("collective risk") being the expected number of cases in an exposed population.

Risk estimation (quantification) is a complex enterprise that has to combine information from, besides exposure assessment, both disease-epidemiological studies and experiments. Due to the low power of epidemiological investigations, it has become a consensus that cancer risks are best estimated from long-term animal experiments. Since in the latter, high doses are required for informative observations to be obtained, the risk estimation involves extrapolations from animal to man and from high to low doses (Hogan & Hoel,1982).

However, these two extrapolations, which are required for risk estimation in human populations, are fraught with difficulties. The extrapolation from high to low doses requires detailed knowledge about the mechanisms at work for a particular substance, and a mathematical model that validly represents these mechanisms over the dose range of interest. The extrapolation from animals to man has several difficulties; one of the main ones, which will also be discussed in the modelling section of this paper, is that carcinogens, according to current understanding, may exercise either a genotoxic effect, i.e., inducing a fundamental mutation in the DNA of a cell, or a promotive effect, i.e., helping a previously induced cell on its way to cancer, or both. In the human population, there are several, both natural and artificial, concurrent causes of initiation and promotion. The effects of a studied substance should therefore be evaluated "on top of the background". An informative animal experiment should, accordingly, be performed at conditions reflecting the variation and other factors present in the human population. This is usually not the case, since experimental animals are genetically similar, live in a pure environment, and are exposed to one substance at a time.

We therefore believe that animal experiments, at present, cannot be considered a reliable source of information for risk estimation for humans. A similar view has recently been expressed by Ames and Gold (1990), who argue that the results of animal cancer tests often are dominated by the promotive effects at high doses, and that these do not reflect the mechanisms at low doses. A more promising method, at least for substances with a genotoxic action, is represented by the"rad-equivalence" approach which, by using γ-radiation as a reference standard for chemical dose, permits an implicit estimation of the background promotive events in a human population (cf. Wright et al.,1989; Ehrenberg,1979,1980). This approach is based on the observation that, at low doses, the γ-radiation dose producing the same forward mutation frequency as a unit of chemical dose, is approximately the same in very different biological systems, most probably including man (Ehrenberg,1979; Kolman et al.,1988). The cancer risk increment from a chemical could, according to this approach, be estimated from

$$P_{can}(D) - P_{can}(0) \approx k_{rad} \times Q \times D,$$

where k_{rad} is the relatively well-defined risk coefficient (in rad^{-1}) for radiogenic cancer, Q a quality factor (in rad $\times$ mMh^{-1}), describing the relative genotoxic effectiveness of a studied chemical, and D the target dose (in mMh) of the chemical. The promotive background in a human population does not have to be estimated separately, since its effects are already included in k_{rad}.

Animal experiments, on the other hand, if properly analyzed, can provide a lot of qualitative information on the mechanisms of carcinogenic action of chemicals. This is especially true if the experiments are approached in a more data-analytical fashion, where certain dose-response curve shapes can be thought of as corresponding to certain main mechanisms of action, several data sets are analyzed and compared, and where conclusions are mainly drawn for the purpose of generating hypotheses and discussion.

In the present report, we summarize certain conclusions from a study of dose-response models fitted to long-term animal experiments, carried out within the work of the Swedish Governmental Committee on Cancer Prevention (1984). In that study, several mathematical models were fitted to published dose-response data for experimental cancer, in all some 100 data sets (von Bahr et al.,1984). A somewhat updated version of details of procedure and results is also available (Scalia-Tomba et al.,1990).

Models and model fitting

Data for long-term chemical cancer tests (published before 1981), with at least four doses, were collected. Thirteen mathematical models (see Table 1) were fitted to these data.

Table 1 Studied models

Code numbers and names	Dose-response function and definition of parameters
1 Probit	$P(D) = \Phi(\alpha + \beta D)$
2 Probit extra	$P(D) = (1 - \gamma) + \gamma\Phi(\alpha + \beta D)$
3 Probit-log	$P(D) = \Phi(\alpha + \beta \log(D))$
4 Logit	$P(D) = \dfrac{1}{(1 + e^{-(\alpha + \beta D)})}$
5 Logit-log	$P(D) = \dfrac{D^{\alpha}}{(D^{\alpha} + \beta^{\alpha})}$
6 One-hit	$P(D) = 1 - e^{-\alpha D}$
7 Armitage-Doll 1	$P(D) = 1 - e^{-(\alpha + \beta D)}$
8 Armitage-Doll 2	$P(D) = 1 - e^{-(\alpha + \beta D + \gamma D^2)}$
9 Cornfield	$P(D) = 1 - e^{-\alpha D/(\beta + D)}$

10 Cornfield extra $P(D) = 1 - e^{-(\alpha + \beta D/(\gamma + D))}$

11 Multi-hit $P(D) = \int_0^D \alpha^\beta \Gamma(\beta)^{-1} x^{\beta-1} e^{-\alpha x} dx$

12 Mixed two-stage $P(D) = (1 - e^{-\gamma D})\Phi(\alpha + \beta D)$

13 Mixed two-stage extra $P(D) = (1 - e^{-(\gamma + \delta D)})\Phi(\alpha + \beta D)$

Eleven of the models (nos. 1-11) are, in principle, of types suggested for extrapolation to low doses. In addition, two multiplicative two-stage models for initiation and promotion are introduced (no. 12 without and no. 13 with background initiation), according to the model

$$P_{can}(D) = P_{ini}(D) \times P_{pro}(D) .$$

This formula represents, in a simplistic way, what was said above about animal experiments, viz. that, in contrast to the situation prevailing in human populations, in animal experiments compounds, at least if no background promotion is present, have to act as complete carcinogens, i.e., provide both initiation and promotion. In these models, the initiation step was described by the one-hit function (nos. 6 and 7, respectively), and for promotion the probit function, i.e. the cumulative normal distribution (no. 2), was chosen (see Fig. 1). Since these models, in contrast to many other multistage (or multihit) models, thus contain one probabilistic and one deterministic (in the sense of describing the distribution of a sensitivity threshold) factor, they were given the working name "mixed two-stage models".

The choice of the probit function for promotion (including cocarcinogenic effects) was based on the assumption that the reprogramming and growth stimulation involved in promotion are associated with a reparative growth appearing particularly at higher doses as a consequence of cytotoxic effects. The probit function has been used to describe radiation death (Grahn,1958). Later studies (Ewing et al.,1988) of the dose-response relationship for the classical promotor 12-O-tetradecanoylphorbol-13-acetate (TPA) also support the choice of the probit function. Besides that, it is difficult to discriminate between the normal distribution and other S-shaped distributions in the range of incidences, 10-90%, where informative observations can usually be obtained.

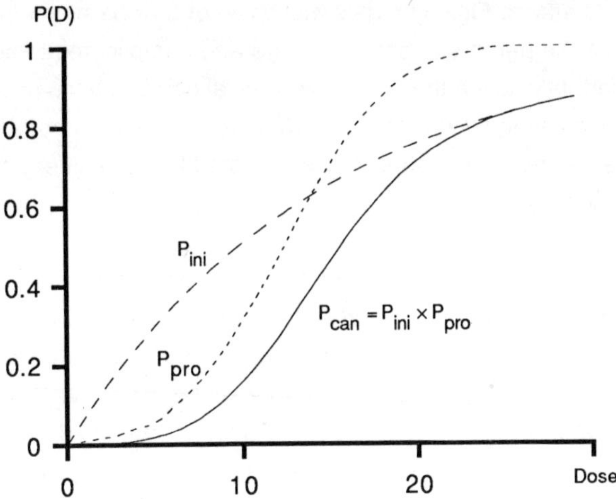

Figure 1 Components of the mixed two-stage model (dose in arbitrary units).

Model fitting

In the models, D expresses the dose of carcinogen or precarcinogen administered according to study protocol. As a rule, the same time scheme is followed for the different doses in an experiment, and the administered (and absorbed) dose will then be proportional to the concentration in food, drinking water, air or solution applied to the skin. For each administered dose D of a given substance, the response is assumed to be binomially distributed with parameters N = no. of exposed or tested animals and p = P(D), according to the model under study. P is a function of dose and of a number of parameters α, β, γ ... (see Table 1). The parameters are fitted using the method of maximum likelihood. The precision of these estimates can be expressed in terms of estimated standard deviations (e.s.d.) or confidence intervals. Since exact mathematical results for the studied models are very difficult to obtain, e.s.d.:s have been calculated using the classical asymptotic theory for maximum likelihood estimators. Furthermore, it is possible to assess the fit of each model to the data set, using the theory of maximum likelihood ratio tests. Thus, for a given data set, a P-value has been calculated for each model, with high values indicating a reasonable fit to data (we will also say that the model is adaptable to data). As in usual significance testing, low P-values indicate that the model should be rejected as a plausible description of the observed data.

Generally speaking, it is easier to fit models with many parameters to a given data set than models with fewer parameters. It is therefore not surprising that models 2, 8, 10, 12 and 13 often seem to fit data better than the models with fewer parameters (although the calculated P-values contain a correction for this effect). Fitting models with three or four parameters often implies numerical problems, since the parameter space is large and complicated to search through and, perhaps more importantly, since there may be several combinations of parameter values giving approximately equally good fits to data. This latter effect often results in large e.s.d.:s for the parameters concerned.It should also be noted that the different parameter estimates in a model are usually correlated.

A general comment on the selection of models is warranted. As stated by Crump (1979), it is highly desirable to introduce into the mathematical models biological functions that are known to affect dose-response relationships. Dose-response curves which are convex (from below) in the low-medium range of doses are very common. This curve shape may have several mechanisms. Besides a promotive action, alone (as in models 1-5) or combined with initiator action (models 12,13), and a genotoxic effect following two-hit kinetics (models 8,11), other, cocarcinogenic, effects may result in similar curve shapes, such as induction of bioactivating enzymes, saturation of enzymes for detoxification of reactive compounds or metabolites, or saturation of DNA repair. For two reasons, it was at this stage not tried to introduce specific functions for such phenomena: the increase of e.s.d. with increasing numbers of variables, and the difficulties in data sets from experiments with small numbers of animals to discriminate between models that may be fitted to convex curves. The drop of the incidence sometimes observed at the highest doses, which has been ascribed to cell killing, was not studied as such. In some instances model fitting was tried with exclusion of such points.

Results

For each analysed data set, the computer program used presents P-values for the fitted models, estimated parameter values with respective e.s.d.:s, estimated values of P(0) and P'(0) (the initial linear slope) with respective e.s.d.:s, comparisons between observations and values expected according to the fitted models, as well as graphical displays of data and fitted models.

From the very large amount of data generated in the study, only a few points of general interest to risk estimation are commented upon in this communication (for details, see Scalia-Tomba et al. (1990); unpublished results may be obtained upon request from the authors). In order to keep notation as compact as possible, sources of data have been numbered and collected in a separate reference list; the numbering is identical to the one used in Scalia-Tomba et al. (1990). In the text, they will be refered to by their number, prefixed with a D. In Tables 2 and 3, examples of results of model fitting to a few data sets of reasonable size are given, followed by brief discussions of each compound.

Table 2 Fit of models to cancer tests with AAF (D135), urethan (D154-157) and vinyl chloride (D120,123). Only models without the requirement P(0) = 0 are included. For each model, the P-values for goodness-of-fit are given (in %). Values below, e.g., 5% can be interpreted as a "bad fit".

Data	Models 1	2	4	7	8	10	13
AAF							
Mouse, Bladder							
18 months	0	41	0	0	0	0	0
24 months	0	66	2	0	0	0	0
Mouse, Liver							
18 months	75	63	61	5	81	3	59
24 months	4	2	0	1	94	0	22
Urethan							
Mouse, all sites	1	0	1	2	1	55	49
Rat, all sites	44	26	41	70	49	49	78
Vinyl chloride							
Rat, 50-10000 ppm, all sites							
60 animals/dose	0	0	0	0	0	83	83
30 animals/dose	32	21	20	33	22	22	13

N-Acetyl-2-aminofluorene (AAF)

The experiment with AAF (D135) is one of the largest animal cancer experiments ever conducted (more than 24000 mice over 8 doses). The table shows the models' fit to data for observed incidences at both 18 and 24 months, the liver data for 18 months being less discriminative because of lower number of observed tumours. As shown in Fig. 2, incidences of bladder tumours exhibit an apparent threshold followed by an upwards bending that singles out the probit model with background incidence (Table 1 no. 2) as the only one that is accepted. This would be the expected curve if the promotion component, $P_{pro}(D)$, is rate-limiting, as it would be if initiation is redundant already at the lowest dose or due to endogenous factors. In fact, levels of DNA adducts (Beland,1990) show that the bladder dose, although lower than the dose in liver cells, is considerable already at the lowest dose.

For liver cancer, several models can be fitted to the 18 months observations, but only the mixed two-stage model (no. 13) and the linear-quadratic model (no. 8) are accepted by the 24 months data. This is in agreement with an upwards bend at higher doses of a nearly linear dose-response curve (see Fig. 2). This bend coincides with a shortening of latency times (Farmer et al.,1980), in compatibility with a superimposed promotive action.

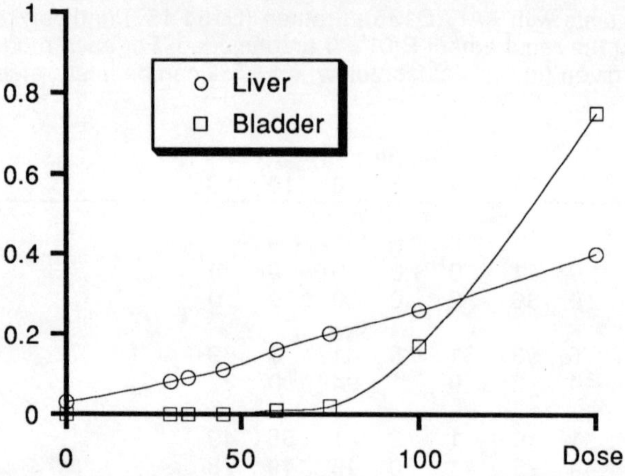

Figure 2 Incidences of liver and bladder tumours after administration of AAF to mice for 24 months. Data from Littlefield et al. (D135).

Urethan

Due to its occurrence in fermented foods (Ough,1976), urethan which was early described as a multipotential carcinogen (Tannenbaum,1964; Mirvish,1968), is a possible cause of cancer in man. The identity of the reactive intermediate(s) of urethan (ethyl carbamate) has long appeared enigmatic. Some support for N-oxygenation to a carbethoxylating species has been obtained (Boyland & Williams,1969) but later data are in favour of a pathway leading to epoxyethyl carbamate (Ribovich et al.,1982). This metabolite will introduce 2-oxoethyl groups on nucleophilic atoms, i.e. the same chemical endpoint as for vinyl chloride (cf. Svensson,1988).

Given in Table 2 are the results of model fitting to the test data of Schmähl et al. (D154-157). Whereas the low incidences in rats did not permit discrimination between models, models no. 10 (for saturation kinetics of bioactivation) and no. 13 (mixed two-stage) were distinctly preferred for the mouse data. In Svensson's (1988) later dosimetric studies, no indication of Michaelis-Menten kinetics was obtained, the levels of oxoethylations in hemoglobin and DNA being linearly related to administered dose. This should be taken to rule out model no. 10 as a correct description of events. The good fit of model no. 13 is compatible with data indicating that urethan may act as initiator (D116,117), as well as promotor (D118,119); see further Scalia-Tomba et al. (1990). A remaining problem is caused by the fact that the promotor function generated by model no. 13 becomes restricted to about one half of the animals, a situation that would be obtained in case of a great variation between animals in sensitivity. A role of the intestinal flora in bioactivation can be excluded (Svensson et al.,1990).

Vinyl chloride

Maltoni's studies of vinyl chloride (D120,123), a carcinogenic pollutant particularly in certain work environments, are of sufficient scope to render analyses of dose-response relationships meaningful. This compound exhibits the same spectrum of preferred models as urethan, models no. 10 and 13 being the only ones accepted by incidence data at 60 animals per dose. The table also illustrates that data for 30 animals per dose were insufficient to discriminate between models. In contrast to the urethan case (see above), the pharmacokinetic model no. 10 seems to describe correctly the saturation kinetics of bioactivation observed in pharmacokinetic studies (Gehring et al.,1978). These kinetics to the reactive intermediate, chloroethylene oxide, which like the one of urethan is oxoethylating (Osterman-Golkar et al.,1977), thus seems to be the incidence limiting factor. This conclusion is strengthened by compatibility of the values of K_m with the biochemically determined value (see Scalia-Tomba et al.,1990). The inclusion of Maltoni's data for 1-25 ppm induces no change of the picture although these data, per se, indicate a somewhat steeper slope at low doses.

The model is further supported by the agreement of the initial slope with the one obtained in a study where vinyl chloride was given by stomach sond. The parameters of the fitted two-stage model describe a rapidly growing promotor effect superimposed on a fairly constant initiation frequency. Although this result appears somewhat unrealistic, it might give a signal that a two-stage model including the saturation kinetics would give a more realistic description. In order to limit the number of parameters, this could only be done with preset values for K_m or tissue doses (Anderson et al.,1980).

Benzo[a]pyrene (BaP)

Several experiments with skin application and observation of local skin sarcomas have been carried out with BaP. In 15 data sets, the number of doses was at least four (D25-27,31-41,43). The fitting of the studied models to these data sets, excluding three the quality of which was such that any model was accepted (D26,35,38), is illustrated in Table 3 by median values and ranges of P-values.

Only the mixed two-stage models can be generally fitted to these data sets ($P > 5\%$). Also the probit-log dose model (no. 3) is rejected in a majority of cases, including data upon which this model was originally developed by Mantel and Bryan (1961) and Mantel and Schneiderman (1975).

Table 3 Fit of the 13 models (see Table 1) to experimental dose-response data for local tumours after skin application of BaP. Medians and ranges of P-values are given for each model. Out of 15 data sets analysed (D25-27,31-41,43), 3 were excluded because they accepted all models (D26,35,38). Models 12 and 13 were pooled because the latter, with 5 parameters, was not always applicable.

Model number (see Table 1)	Values of P for model fit: Median	Range
1	0	0-36
2	0	0-23
3	3	0-72
4	0	0-21
5	2	0-87
6	0	0-58
7	0	0-44
8	0	0-48
9	0	0-84
10	0	0-55
11	1	0-51
12, 13	25 (47[a])	7-74 (7-75[a])

[a] All 15 data sets

Also in several other data sets, among others for methylcholanthrene, these two-stage models are preferred.

In the study of Payne and Hueper (D41,43), dose-response curves for BaP were determined at 7 doses (including control), administered subcutaneously either as single doses or as 12 fractions given with one month intervals.The fractionated treatments lead to a higher incidence at higher doses than the single treatments (see Fig. 3), indicating a saturation of metabolism in the latter case.

In agreement herewith also the pharmaco-kinetic model (no. 10; cf Table 4) was adaptable to the single dose experiments, but not to the one with fractionated doses. The value of $\alpha \approx 0$ in the Φ-function of model 13 suggests that already the lowest dose has a certain promotive action, with a relatively high value of P'(0). In contrast, for the fractionated doses, $\alpha = -2.5$, corresponding to $P_{pro}(0) \approx 0.01$, and a slope P'(0) that is more than 10 times less than the one of the single dose experiment. However, for the two experiments, the values of the coefficients for initiation, δ in no. 13 and β in no. 10, are of the same magnitude in the different models. This exemplifies that parameter values of the initiation and promotion functions generated are reasonable.

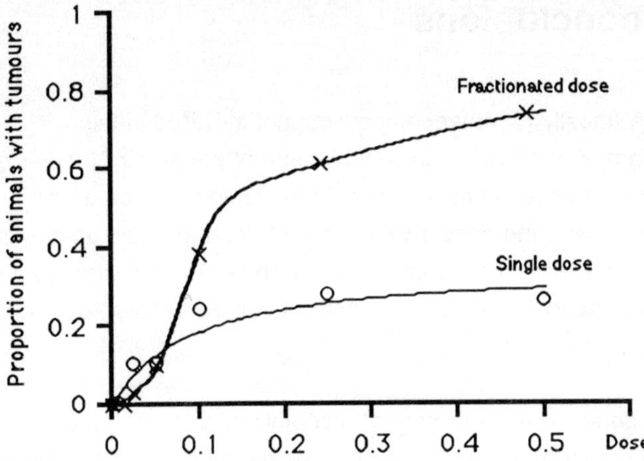

Figure 3 Effect of fractionation on the dose response relationship for BaP. Data from Payne and Hueper (D41,43).

Table 4 BaP. Influence of fractionation of doses on parameter values (± e.s.d) in the pharmaco-kinetical and two-stage models (D41 = single dose, D43 = fractionated dose).

	Model formula				P'(0)	Fit (P-value in %)
Model 10	$P(D) = 1 - e^{-(\alpha + \beta D/(1 + \gamma D))}$					
	α	β	γ			
Single	0	3.9±1.3	8.9±4.6		3.9±1.3	14
Fract.	0	3.3±0.6	0.14±0.6		3.3±0.6	0
Model 13	$P(D) = (1 - e^{-(\gamma + \delta D)})\Phi(\alpha + \beta D)$					
	γ	δ	α	β		
Single	0	6.7±7.7	-0.1±1.1	.-1.0±2.1	3.1±0.9	14
Fract.	0.55±0.33	1.6±1.0	-2.5±0.3	32.6±7.6	0.23±0.17	58

Discussion and conclusions

The examples given, and data, mostly for other compounds, not included in this communication (see Scalia-Tomba et al.,1990) show that different patterns of models are adaptable to different data sets for experimental cancer. This should be taken as an illustration of different chemicals inducing cancer with different dependences on administered dose, sometimes with an influence also of experimental conditions. A conclusion from this is that no unique model based on theory for action mechanisms can be adapted generally to incidence data from long-term cancer tests.

Adaptable models may be understood as indicators of predominating traits in the dose-response curves, with some likelihood reflecting factors in the mechanisms. For example, for AAF, the preferred models are compatible with promotion (model no. 2) and initiation (no. 8, with a weak quadratic term) being determinants of the incidences of cancer of the bladder and liver, respectively, other effects being possibly redundant already at low doses. In the case of vinyl chloride and several other materials, the saturation of bioactivation, i.e. in principle a one-hit function at low doses, seems to be limiting.

Of particular interest is the broad adaptability of the mixed two-stage models. These models generate functions with reasonable values for initiation, and the parameters for the simultaneously obtained deterministic function can also illustrate to which extent the induced promotive processes are additive to processes that are already ongoing in the animals (Crump et al.,1976). These models also give a unitary description of why initiations (e.g., ionizing radiation (cf. UNSCEAR,1972) and AAF (cf. discussion above)) give rise to tumours sometimes in a linear dependence on dose, i.e., when $P_{pro}(0) \neq 0$, sometimes above an indicated threshold, i.e., when $P_{pro}(0) = 0$, and also of the observed linearization of a threshold curve upon addition of a promotor (Burns et al.,1983). In contrast to animal data for radiogenic cancer (Storer et al.,1988), human epidemiological data for radiation-induced cancer indicate throughout linear dose-responses at low doses (BEIR,1990), as would be expected with a naturally occuring background promotion.

Acknowledgments

This study was supported financially by the Bank of Sweden Tercentenary Foundation (project no. RJ 86/313) and by the US Department of Energy (project no. DE-FG02-89ER60784).

General References

Ames BN, Gold LS (1990) Too many rodent carcinogens: mitogenesis increases mutagenesis. Science 249: 970-971.
Anderson MW, Hoel DG, Kaplan NL (1980) A general scheme for the incorporation of pharmacokinetics in low-dose risk estimation for chemical carcinogenesis: Example - Vinyl chloride. Toxicol Appl Pharmacol 55: 154-161.
BEIR V (1990) Health effects of exposure to low levels of ionizing radiation. National Academy Press, Washington DC.
Beland FA, Fullerton NF, Kinouchi T, Smith BA, Poirier MC (1990) DNA adduct formation in relation to tumorigenesis in mice chronically fed 2-acetylaminofluorene. In: Mouse Liver Carcinogenesis: Mechanisms and Species Comparisons, Alan R. Liss, Inc.: 121-129.
Boyland E, Williams K (1969) Reactions of urethane with nucleic acids in vivo. Biochem J 111: 121-127.
Burns F, Alberg R, Altshuler B, Morris E (1983) Approach to risk assessment for genotoxic carcinogens based on data from the mouse skin initiation-promotion model. Environ Health Persp 50: 309-320.
Crump KS (1979) Dose response problems in carcinogenesis. Biometrics 35: 157-167.
Crump KS, Hoel DG, Langley CH, Peto R (1976) Fundamental carcinogenic processes and their implications for low dose risk assessment. Cancer Res 36: 2973-2979.
Ehrenberg L (1979) Risk assessment of ethylene oxide and other compounds. In McElheny VK, Abrahamson S (eds.), Assessing Chemical Mutagens: The risk to Humans (Banbury Rep No 1), CSH Press, Cold Spring Harbor, NY: 157-190.
Ehrenberg L (1980) Methods of comparing risks of radiation and chemicals. In: Radiobiological equivalents of chemical pollutants, IAEA, Vienna: 11-21, 23-36.
Ehrenberg L, Moustacchi E, Osterman-Golkar S, with an Appendix by Ekman G (1983) Dosimetry of genotoxic agents and dose-response relationships of their effects. Mutat Res 123: 121-182.
Ewing MW, Conti CJ, Kruszewski FH, Slaga TJ, DiGiovanni J (1988) Tumor progression in sencar mouse skin as a function of initiator dose and promoter dose, duration, and type. Cancer Res 48: 7048-7054.
Farmer JH, Kodell RL, Greenman DL (1980) Dose and time response models for the incidence of bladder and liver neoplasms in mice fed 2-acetylaminofluorene continuosly. J Environ Pathol Toxicol 3: 55-68.
Gehring PJ, Watanabe PG, Park CN (1978) Resolution of dose-response toxicity data for chemicals requiring metabolic activation: example - vinyl chloride. Toxicology and Appl Pharmacol 44: 581-591.
Grahn D (1958) Acute radiation response of mice from a cross between radiosensitive and radioresistant strains. Genetics 43: 835-843.
Hogan MD, Hoel DG (1982) Extrapolation to man. In: Haynes AW (Ed.) Principles and Methods of Toxicology, Raven Press, New York, 711-730.
Kolman A, Segerbäck D, Osterman-Golkar S (1988) Estimation of the cancer risk of genotoxic chemicals by the rad-equivalence approach. IARC Sci Publ 89: 258-264.
Mantel N, Bryan WR (1961) Safety testing of carcinogenic agents. J Nat Cancer Inst 27: 455-570.
Mantel N, Schneiderman MA (1975) Estimating "safe" levels, a hazardous undertaking. Cancer Res 38: 1379-1386.
Mirvish SS (1968) The carcinogenic action and metabolism of urethan and N-hydroxyurethan. Adv Cancer Res 11: 1-42.
O'Riordan T (1979) Environmental impact analyses and risk assessment in a management perspective. In: Goodman GT, Rowe WD (eds.), Energy Risk Management, Academic Press, New York: 21-36.
Osterman-Golkar S, Hultmark D, Segerbäck D, Calleman CJ, Göthe R, Ehrenberg L, Wachtmeister CA (1977) Alkylation of DNA and proteins in mice exposed to vinyl chloride. Biochem Biophys Res Commun 76: 259-266.

Ough CS (1976) Ethyl carbamate in fermented beverages and foods. I. Naturally occuring ethyl carbamate. J Agr Food Chem 24:323-327.
Ribovich ML, Miller JA, Miller EC, Timmins LG (1982) Labeled 1,$\underline{N}^6$-ethenoadenosine and 3,$\underline{N}^4$-ethenocytidine in hepatic RNA of mice given ethyl-1,2-^{3}H or ethyl-1-^{14}C ethyl carbamate (urethan). Carcinogenesis 3: 539-546.
Scalia-Tomba G, von Bahr B, Säfwenberg J-O, Ehrenberg L (1990) Mathematical extrapolation models in cancer risk assessment. Technical rep B:12, Dept Math Stat, Stockholm University, Sweden.
Storer JB, Mitchell TJ, Fry RJM (1988) Extrapolation of the relative risk of radiogenic neoplasms across mouse strains and to man. Radiat Res 114: 331-353.
Svensson K (1988) Alkylation of protein and DNA in mice treated with urethane. Carcinogenesis 9: 2197-2201.
Svensson K et al. (1990) To be published.
Swedish Governmental Committee on Cancer Prevention (1984) Cancer; Causes, prevention, etc.. Swedish Government Official Report 1984:67, Stockholm.
Tannenbaum A (1964) Contributions of urethan studies to the understanding of carcinogenesis. National Cancer Institute Monograph 14: 341-356.
UNSCEAR, United Nations Committee on the Effects of Atomic Radiation (1972) Ionizing Radiation: Levels and Effects, Vol. II: Effects. Report to the General Assembly, United Nations, New York.
von Bahr B, Ehrenberg L, Scalia-Tomba G ,Säfwenberg J-O (1984) Study of different models for dose-response relationships (in Swedish). Appendix 9, Report to the Governmental Committee on Cancer Prevention, Ds S 1984:5, Stockholm.
Wright AS, Bradshaw TK, Watson WP (1989) Prospective detection and assessment of genotoxic hazards: A critical appreciation of the contribution of L.G. Ehrenberg. IARC Sci Publ 89: 237-248.

References to analysed data sets

	Data set number
N-acetylaminofluorene (AAF)	
Littlefield NA et al.(1980) Environ Pathol Toxicol 3 (Special issue 3):17.	135
Benzo[a]pyrene	
Poel WE (1963) Nat Cancer Inst Monogr 10: 611.	25-30
Roe FJC et al. (1970) Brit J Cancer 24: 788.	31
Bingham E, Falk HL (1969) Arch Environ Health 19: 779.	32
Poel WE (1959) J Nat Cancer Inst 22: 19.	33
Wynder EL et al. (1960) Cancer 13: 106.	34,35
Bryan WR, Shimkin MB (1943) J Nat Cancer Inst 3: 503.	36
Hieger I (1959) Brit J Cancer 13: 439.	37
Oberling C et al. (1939) Bull Ass Franc Cancer 28: 198.	38
Rivière MR et al. (1963) Bull Ass Franc Cancer 50: 275.	39
Leiter J, Shear MJ (1943) J Nat Cancer Inst 3: 455.	40
Payne WW, Hueper WC (1960) Am Ind Hyg Ass J 21: 350.	41-43
Urethan	
Berenblum I, Haran-Ghera N (1957) Brit J Cancer 11: 77.	116,117
Vesselinovich SD, Mihailovich N (1966) Cancer Res 26: 1633.	118,119
Schmähl D et al. (1977) Int J Cancer 19: 77.	154-157
Vinyl chloride	
Maltoni C et al. (1974) Med Lav 65: 421.	120
Maltoni C (1977) In: Hiatt et al. (eds.9), Origins of Human Cancer, Book A, Cold Spring Harbor: 119.	121,123

STATISTICAL PROBLEMS IN ESTIMATING A THRESHOLD IN A DOSE-RESPONSE MODEL

Fredrik Granath
Dept. of Mathematical Statistics
Stockholm University, Sweden

Introduction

In risk assessment, dose-response curves for mutation and cancer induced by genotoxic agents are usually assumed to be linear at low doses (ICRP, 1977; Ehrenberg et al.,1983). However, the true shape of the dose-response curves for mutation and cancer at very low doses has been debated; e.g., the question of the existence or non-existence of a no-effect threshold is a subject of opposing opinions. This is partly a consequence of the fact that, for statistical reasons, there is always a detection limit below which informative observations are not obtainable. Deviations from linearity could occur, e.g., if there are inducible functions that affect the response to genotoxic agents. A settling of this problem would lead to a more realistic debate concerning risk assessment and a better basis for decision making.

The objective of this work is to find methods to assess the information value of available data with respect to the existence of thresholds. The general idea of the method to be presented is to judge, based on an estimate of the background risk, whether the incidence at low doses is compatible with a threshold or with the model at higher doses.
Two basic assumptions must be fulfilled:

- For the higher doses there is a biologically reasonable "extrapolation" model with a linear component.
- An estimate of the background risk is available.

Statistical Method

The data collected from a typical experiment of the type studied here is the following: At each of a number of doses, $D_1,D_2,....,D_k$, a number of experimental units, $n_1,n_2,....,n_k$, are exposed and a dichotomous outcome is observed. The chosen model is the simplest one that has a no-effect threshold: a piecewise defined model with constant risk up to the threshold dose, and for higher doses a linear increase with increasing dose. The advantage of this model is that it has the nice property that the threshold dose is an explicit parameter. This can be formalized as follows: Independent random variables, $X_1, X_2, \ldots, X_k$, are observed, where $X_i \sim Bin(n_i, p_i)$. The dose-response curve, p(D), can be parametrized in the following ways:

$$p(D) = \alpha + \beta(D-\gamma)^+ \quad \text{, where } (z)^+ = \max(0,z) \text{ ,}$$

or, alternatively,

$$p(D) = \begin{cases} A_1 & \text{if } D < \gamma \\ A_2 + BD & \text{if } D \geq \gamma \end{cases} \quad \text{, with the restriction} \quad \gamma = \frac{A_1 - A_2}{B} \text{ .}$$

The problem is now to estimate the parameters of this model and to derive goodness of fit tests and hypothesis tests. This problem has been treated in earlier studies, in the situation with regression on normally distributed observations; a thorough investigation of this topic is given by Feder (1974). There are a couple of unusual features of this kind of piecewise defined model making it different from regression problems having the same parametric form of the regression function through the entire observed dose range.

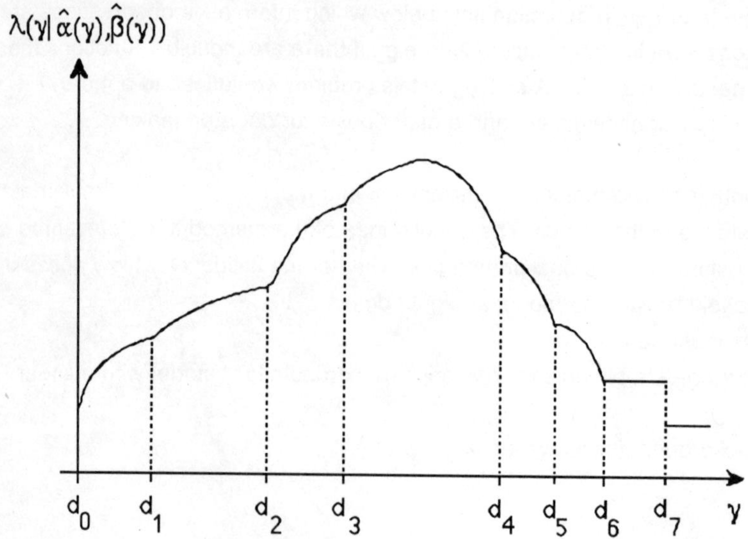

Figure 1 *The principal shape of the profile log-likelihood function of* γ.

Classical maximum likelihood (ML) theory, see e.g., Rao (1965), assumes the likelihood to be a differentiable function in the neighbourhood of the true parameter value. Figure 1 shows that this is not the case for the proposed model when the shiftpoint γ coincides with a dose point. This implies that results such as asymptotic normality of the ML-estimator cannot be expected in such a situation. The figure also illustrates another unusual feature concerning the identifiability of the parameters; the likelihood is flat for $\gamma > d_{k-1}$. In this parameter region the design does not allow identification of the parameters of the model. The design has to be such that at least one dose point lies in the dose range of the constant segment and two lie in the linear segment. This generally requires some kind of a priori knowledge about the location of the threshold parameter. Typically this is not a problem, at least not in trials with known carcinogens or mutagens. Then the control dose represents the constant segment, if any, and at high doses there is an increased risk.

Results

The results presented below are asymptotic, i.e., valid for the situation where the number of experimental units n_i at each dose d_i tends to infinity. In a forthcoming paper (Granath, 1990), it is shown that the asymptotic distribution of the ML-estimator depends on whether the true threshold parameter γ^0 coincides with a dose point or not, as follows:

CASE 1 : $d_i \neq \gamma^0$
All regularity conditions for applying classical ML theory are fulfilled and it can be shown that
$\sqrt{n}\,(\hat{\theta} - \theta^0) \overset{as}{\sim} N(0,Q^{-1})$,
where θ *denotes the vector* (α,β,γ) *and Q is the information matrix.*

CASE 2: $d_i = \gamma^0$
The asymptotic distribution becomes a mixture of two different normal distributions and a point mass in $\{d_i = \gamma^0\}$.

Consequences of this result on the inference concerning γ

Estimation procedure: the likelihood function of γ may be multimodal or attain its maximum at a design point. Therefore, thorough examination of the profile likelihood of γ is needed. Each possible partition of data points into the constant risk and increasing risk segments has to be investigated. For a more complete discussion of the estimation procedure, see Hinkley (1971).

Testing hypotheses: a likelihood ratio test, using the critical levels of a chi square distribution, is recommended. Tests based on the assumed asymptotic normal distribution of the ML-estimator should be avoided because they can be misleading unless data gives precise information on the location of γ.

Confidence intervals: construction of confidence intervals from inversion of the likelihood ratio test is recommended, i. e., the confidence interval includes all values γ^0 that cannot be rejected in a likelihood ratio test of $\hat{\gamma} = \gamma^0$. Intervals constructed assuming an asymptotic normal distribution of the ML-estimator should be avoided for the same reasons as given above.

Example 1: Mutagenicity of X-rays on *Tradescantia* stamen hairs (data from Sparrow et al. 1972).

This is an example of the application of the above described method, a brief analysis of a dose response experiment where stamen hairs of *Tradescantia* were exposed to X-rays and frequencies of pink-mutant events of *Tradescantia* clone 0.2 were observed. This is a very large binomial experiment which seems suitable for this kind of analysis.

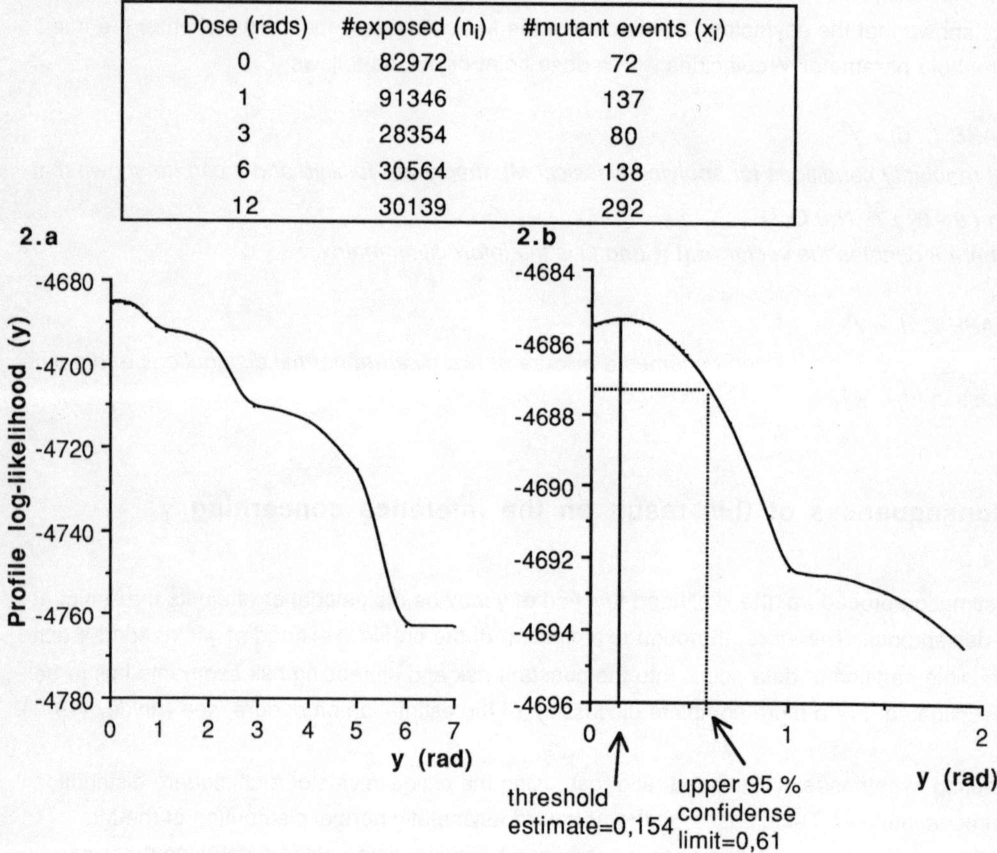

Dose (rads)	#exposed (n_i)	#mutant events (x_i)
0	82972	72
1	91346	137
3	28354	80
6	30564	138
12	30139	292

Figure 2 *Figure 2.a shows the entire profile log-likelihood function of the threshold parameter. Figure 2.b shows the confidence interval of threshold parameter constructed from inversion of likelihood ratio tests.*

When fitting the model with a threshold (i.e. $p_i = \alpha + \beta(d_i-\gamma)^+$), the ML-estimates of the parameters are $\hat{\alpha} = 8.7 \cdot 10^{-4}$, $\hat{\beta} = 7.1 \cdot 10^{-4}$, $\hat{\gamma} = 0.16$. The value of the goodness of fit statistic $T_1 = 2.20$, and, since T_1 is $\chi^2(2)$ distributed under the hypothesis $H_1 : \gamma > 0$, there are no signs of a bad fit. For testing the hypothesis $H_0 : \gamma = 0$, the corresponding goodness of fit statistic $T_0 = 2.58$ is calculated. H_0 is then rejected if the difference T_0-T_1 is too large. The distribution of T_0-T_1 under H_0 is a 50:50 mixture of a point mass in {0} and a $\chi^2(1)$ distribution. This implies that $Pr(T_0-T_1 > 0.38) = 0.25$. Hence H_0 cannot be rejected; i.e., the data do not support the existence of a threshold dose (an even larger experiment from Sparrow results in an estimate of no threshold and yields an upper confidence limit of 0.07 rad, corresponding to a mean of about 1 hit/cell nucleus).

Example 2: Mutagenicity of ethylene oxide on *E. coli* (data from Hussain 1984).

The analysis of this data set applies the threshold model to the relative risk compared to the control (i.e., $RR=1+\beta(d_i-\gamma)^+$). The observations have been fitted by weighted least squares, where the weights are the reciprocals of the variance of each observation. This variance has been calculated assuming the Poisson distribution for the number of colonies counted.

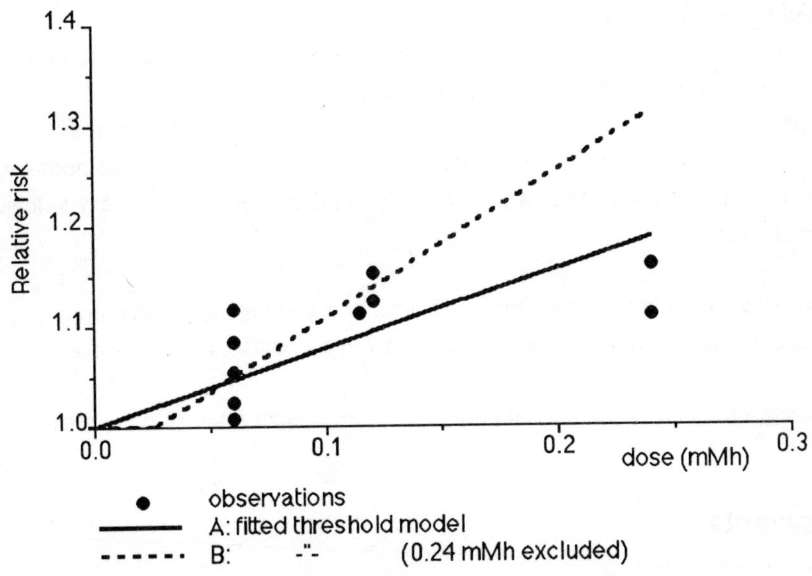

Figure 3 *Threshold model fitted to relative risk*

The threshold parameter is estimated to be zero when the model is applied to the complete data (A in Fig. 3) and the upper confidence limit is as low as 0.025 mMh. The fit is, however, somewhat suspect; it is almost significantly bad ($p \approx 0.10$) and the residuals seem to be systematic. Excluding the dose 0.24 mMh, the data was fitted to the model again (B in Fig. 3). This results in a more reasonable fit, with an estimated threshold of 0.03 mMh ($p \approx 0.13$), and yields an upper confidence limit of 0.05 mMh. This dose corresponds to a mean of 0.2 hits/cell nucleus, alkylations of guanine-$\underline{O}^6$ in DNA being considered as hits. The relative risks for the two 0.24 mMh points now both deviate significantly from the values predicted by the model fitted to the doses 0.06 and 0.12 mMh. The conclusion from these analyses is that data support a theory of super-linearity rather than sub-linearity in the low-dose region.

Comment: this example shows that the conclusions can be strongly dependent on model choice. For instance, the narrow confidence interval reflects the bad fit of the model, in the sense that, if the intercept had been a free parameter, it would have been estimated to be larger than 1, but this contradicts the assumption of the model, since the relative risk at dose zero is 1 by definition.

Conclusions

1. A significant threshold parameter implies the existence of a threshold in the sense that the slope of the dose-response curve, in some dose interval at low doses, is smaller than the slope indicated by the model at higher doses.

• If a threshold is found, there is reason to look for additional mechanisms causing such a shape (cf. Ehrenberg et al. 1983), e.g., inducible systems for error-prone repair.

• It must be noted that a significant threshold as well as a very small upper limit of a confidence interval for the threshold can be caused by a misspecification of the model at higher doses. This stresses the need for testing the fit of the model and especially to look out for systematic residuals.

2. A confidence interval provides a lower and upper limit of the threshold parameter.

• Data of good quality may provide an upper limit too low to be considered as biologically reasonable.

• A wide confidence interval reflects that data are uninformative with respect to the model.

Acknowledgments

This work was carried out in collaboration with the Dept. of Radiobiology at Stockholm University and supported financially by the Bank of Sweden Tercentenary Foundation (project no. RJ 86/313) and by the US Department of Energy (project no. DE-FG02-89ER60784).

References

Ehrenberg L, Moustacchi E, Osterman-Golkar S, with an Appendix by Ekman G (1983) Dosimetry of genotoxic agents and dose-response relationships of their effects. Mutat Res 123: 121-182.

Feder PI (1975) On asymptotic distribution in segmented regression problems – identified case. Ann Stat 3: 49-83.

Granath F (1990) Aspects of hockey stick regression. To be published.

Hinkley DV (1971) Inference in two-phase regression. JASA 66: 736-742.

Hussain S (1984) Dose-response relationship for mutations induced in E. coli by some model compounds. Hereditas 101: 57-68.

ICRP, International Commission on Radiological Protection (1977) Recommendations (Publ 26), Pergamon Press,Oxford.

Rao CR (1965) Linear statistical inference. Wiley, New York.

Sparrow AH, Underbrink AG , Rossi HH (1972) Mutation induced in Tradescantia by small doses of X-rays and neutrons: Analysis of dose-response curves. Science 176: 916-918.

PER-LITTER ANALYSES FOR STUDIES OF DEVELOPMENTAL TOXICITY

Walter W. Piegorsch and Joseph K. Haseman
Statistics and Biomathematics Branch
National Institute of Environmental Health Sciences
Research Triangle Park, NC 27709, U.S.A.

Introduction

An important concern in statistical analyses of developmental toxicity studies involves evaluation of the teratogenic or heritable mutagenic potential of the experimental stimulus. If the experimental design is directed at analysis of pre-natal malformations, deaths, or other detrimental characteristics incurred by the fetus after *in utero* exposure (McLachlan et al., 1987), the endpoint is by nature teratogenic (Gad and Weil, 1986, §11; Manson and Kang, 1989). Alternatively, if the experimental design is directed at identification of developmental damage to the gametes, resulting in toxic effects passed on from parent to offspring, the endpoint is a (heritable) genotoxic one. An example of such a genotoxicity assay is the Dominant Lethal test performed with male mice (Epstein et al., 1972; Ehling et al., 1978).

Of primary concern when analyzing such data is the proper recognition and definition of the experimental unit (EU). Statistically, the EU is regarded as the (largest) sampling unit to which the treatment is applied. For a typical teratogenicity assay, this is the (pregnant) female; for the dominant lethal mutagenicity assay, the EU is usually the male (James and Smith, 1982; Vuataz and Sotek, 1978). For dominant lethal testing, if only one female is mated to one treated male, then the EU may be regarded as the mating pair. Proper definition of the EU is important, since statistical analyses typically suppose that the observations are mutually independent of each other. If the EU is, say, the female, then fetuses sampled from that female represent multiple observations on the individual EU (female) that may be correlated with each other. If this correlation is not taken into account, calculated test statistics or confidence intervals will exhibit increases in their false positive error rates (Haseman and Soares, 1976).

For developmental toxicity assays in rodents, each individual fetus is examined for a toxic response, hence one may be tempted to perform the statistical analysis at a per-fetus level without correcting for possible correlations among the fetal responses (Becker, 1974; Kalter, 1974). Since the EU is clearly the female or mating pair in these cases, one should expect any teratogenic or mutagenic malformations to cluster within litters. The correct approach is to recognize that, as the EU, the female passes along treatment effects to the entire litter. As such, the litter can be alternatively regarded as the EU (Healy, 1972; Khera et al., 1989, Ch. 7; Weil, 1970), resulting in what is termed a *per-litter* analysis of the experimental data (Haseman and Hogan, 1975).

Statistical analyses for discrete response variables

Commonly, the response of interest is discrete, such as number of fetal deaths or malformations. Assume that the index i=1,...,T indicates treatment group (T≥2), which can include a control group at i=1. Within each group, the index j=1,...,J_i indicates each litter; within each litter, k=1,...,n_{ij} indicates individual fetuses. The per-fetus observation is then Y_{ijk}. We will denote the per-litter response as Y_{ij}, and write $L = \sum_{i=1}^{T} J_i$. If the Y_{ij} are taken as number of affected fetuses in the jth litter of the ith treatment group, then the possible values of Y_{ij} are the integers from zero to n_{ij}.

In the discrete case, we caution against proceeding by direct calculations on the Y_{ij}. Unless the n_{ij} are all (approximately) equal, this approach fails to correct for the quantitative effects of differing n_{ij}. Control of this difference is incorporated into the statistical analysis most simply by adjusting the observed counts, Y_{ij}, by their corresponding litter sizes, n_{ij}: $Z_{ij} = Y_{ij}/n_{ij}$. Thus Z_{ij} is the per-litter proportion of affected fetuses. We also note that the n_{ij} are themselves random variables. As such, analyses employing the information in each n_{ij} should constrain their inferences to be conditional on the observed pattern of the n_{ij}. Approaches that correct for this conditionality typically impose some external distributional assumptions on the n_{ij}; we discuss some of these methods below. A model-free alternative to such operations when T=2 involves stratifying the per-litter observations by the observed litter-sizes, and performing a Mantel-Haenszel correction for analysis over the various strata (Paul and Mantel, 1989).

Response variables in the form Y_{ij}/n_{ij} are often analyzed under a binomial assumption on the Y_{ij} with the added assumption that the probability of response, p_i, does not vary within a treatment group. Unfortunately, the binomial distribution has been shown to provide consistently poor fits to both teratogenic (Haseman and Kupper, 1979; Paul, 1982; Shirley and Hickling, 1981) and dominant lethal mutagenic (Aeschbacher et al., 1977; Haseman and Soares, 1976) data. The overdispersion brought about by the intra-litter correlation requires the construction of alternative models and methods for analysis of the treatment effects. Possible approaches are discussed in the following sections.

Distribution-free methods based on ranks

Rank-based methods for assessing possible treatment differences are appropriate under a variety of distributional assumptions (Gad and Weil, 1986, pp.59-69). For this analysis, we assume only that the observed proportions, Z_{ij}, have median values ζ_i (i=1,...,T), where typically ζ_i will be a function of p_i. To test the (null) hypothesis $H_0:\zeta_1=\zeta_2=\cdots=\zeta_T$ versus any difference among the ζ_i, one applies the Kruskal-Wallis test (Gad and Weil, 1986, pp.67-69; Lehmann, 1975, §5.2). An important feature here is that the conditionality on the observed pattern of the n_{ij}'s is not required for this analysis. There is, however, the additional requirement that the *shapes* of the underlying distributions for the Z_{ij} be equivalent. This shape homogeneity may be invalidated when large disparities exist among the n_{ij}. To correct for possible heterogeneity, an alternative formulation that employs an arc-sine (Brier et al., 1986, eq. 4) or angular (Anscombe, 1948) transform of the original values of Y_{ij} and n_{ij} can be utilized.

When testing H_0 against the specific alternative that some monotone increasing relationship exists among the ζ_i, one applies the Jonckheere-Terpstra test for ordered alternatives (Lehmann, 1975, §5.5B). The alternative hypothesis becomes $H_1:\zeta_1\leq\cdots\leq\zeta_T$ (with strict inequality in effect somewhere among the ζ_i). Corrections are recommended if there are a large number of tied observations (Lehmann, 1975, pp.235-236), especially at a single rank value (Haseman and Hoel, 1974; Lin and Haseman, 1976).

Of additional interest are rank-based procedures that (i) test H_0 against an ordered increase that may be contaminated by some downturn at high doses (Simpson and Margolin, 1986), or (ii) simultaneously compare all treatments pairwise, or against a control group (Miller, 1981, §§3.3-3.4)

Resampling approaches for per-litter analyses

Although rank-based methods have been shown empirically to be acceptable for per-litter analyses (Haseman and Soares, 1976; Lamb et al., 1981; Pasternack and Shore, 1982), one concern that is sometimes voiced over their use is their failure to take the magnitude of observed differences among the Z_{ij} into account. Transforming the proportions into ranks — it is argued (Mantel, 1979) — imposes an inappropriate or unreasonable scaling (i.e., the ranks) on the observed scale of measurement where once a reasonable scale (i.e., the proportions) existed. Distribution-free alternatives to rank-based methods that retain the original scale of measurement can involve statistical *resampling* plans. These approaches require no stringent distributional assumptions on the Y_{ij} (such as a binomial sampling assumption); rather, they only require existence of low-order population moments. They then attempt to use the data points themselves to suggest estimators for (functions of) these moments' values.

One such method is known as "jackknifing," originally proposed by Quenouille (1949). Effectively, jackknifing requires the user to specify some form of estimator for the parameter of interest, and then to apply repeatedly that estimator to subsamples of the original data. The application of statistical jackknifing to per-litter analysis is discussed by Gladen (1979). The parameters of interest are the treatment probabilities of affliction, p_i (i=1,...,T). Under the assumption that $E(Y_{ij}|n_{ij}) = n_{ij}p_i$, the estimator $\hat{p}_i = \sum_{j=1}^{J_i} Y_{ij} / \sum_{j=1}^{J_i} n_{ij}$ is unbiased for p_i. A distribution-free jackknife estimator of var($\hat{p}_i$) is

$$s_i^2 = \frac{J_i - 1}{J_i} \sum_{j=1}^{J_i} \left(\hat{p}_{i(j)} - \overline{p}_{i(\cdot)} \right)^2$$

with $\hat{p}_{i(j)} = \sum_{k=1;k\neq j}^{J_i} Y_{ik} / \sum_{k=1;k\neq j}^{J_i} n_{ik}$ and $\overline{p}_{i(\cdot)} = \sum_{j=1}^{J_i} \hat{p}_{i(j)}/J_i$. Under the conditional moment assumptions $E(Y_{ij}|n_{ij}) = n_{ij}p_i$ and $\text{var}(Y_{ij}|n_{ij}) = \tau(n_{ij})$, for some positive-valued function $\tau(\cdot)$, the limiting distribution of $(\hat{p}_i - p_i)/s_i$ is standard normal. A further technical assumption required for this convergence is that, unconditionally, the n_{ij} follow some bounded probability distribution (Gladen, 1979). These results allow for an approximate test of $H_0{:}p_i{=}p_{i'}$ versus $H_1{:}p_i{\neq}p_{i'}$: reject H_0 when the statistic $|\hat{p}_i - \hat{p}_{i'}|/(s_i^2 + s_{i'}^2)^{1/2}$ is larger than an appropriate standard normal quantile, or, to correct for finite sample sizes, a *t*-quantile at $J_i{+}J_{i'}{-}2$ degrees of freedom (Gladen, 1979).

Another form of statistical resampling that has gained recent attention is known as *bootstrap* analysis (Efron, 1982). Bootstrapping employs the empirical distribution of the observed random sample to estimate var($\hat{p}_i$) via many (say, R) simulated resamples of the data. Frangos and Stone (1984) describe a form of bootstrap estimator that has application in per-litter analyses. Simplified, suppose we're given a set of L pairs of observations $\{(Y_{ij},n_{ij})\}_{i=1}^{T}{}_{j=1}^{J_i}$. The empirical distribution of these data places a constant probability mass of 1/L at each data pair. (Recall that $L=\sum_{i=1}^{T} J_i$.) This distribution is then employed to infer qualities of the population from which the sample was originally drawn.

The rth bootstrap resample, $\{(Y_{ij}^{(r)},n_{ij}^{(r)})\}_{i=1}^{T}{}_{j=1}^{J_i}$ (r=1,...,R), yields resample estimates of the p_i:

$$\hat{p}_i^{(r)} = \sum_{j=1}^{J_i} Y_{ij}^{(r)} / \sum_{j=1}^{J_i} n_{ij}^{(r)}$$

(i=1,...,T). After simulating R such random resamples, the bootstrap estimator of var($\hat{p}_i$) is simply $\hat{\text{var}}_R(\hat{p}_i) = \sum_{r=1}^{R} (\hat{p}_i^{(r)} - \overline{p}_i)^2/(R-1)$, where $\overline{p}_i = \sum_{r=1}^{R} \hat{p}_i^{(r)}/R$. With this, large-sample asymptotic normality of $(\hat{p}_i - p_i)/(\hat{\text{var}}_R(\hat{p}_i))^{1/2}$ is often invoked, leading to similar applications and test statistics as those noted for the jackknife estimator, above. Practical values of R can range from 100 to 4000, depending on the application. Carr (1989) presents further uses and improvements of this bootstrapping approach for per-litter analyses.

Generalized parametric linear models

An important generalization of the binomial model is the so-called beta-binomial distribution (Johnson and Kotz, 1969, §9.4). Conditional on n_{ij}, the extra-binomial variability in Y_{ij} is modeled via a beta distribution for the response probabilities: if the ith litter's response probability is given a beta distribution with parameters α_i and β_i (Johnson and Kotz, 1970, §24), the probability that Y_{ij} takes on a value y in the range $\{0,\ldots,n_{ij}\}$ is

$$\Pr[Y_{ij} = y \mid n_{ij}] = \frac{\Gamma(n_{ij}+1)}{\Gamma(y+1)\,\Gamma(n_{ij}-y+1)} \frac{\Gamma(\alpha_i + y)\,\Gamma\left(n_{ij}+\beta_i - y\right)\Gamma(\alpha_i+\beta_i)}{\Gamma(\alpha_i)\,\Gamma(\beta_i)\,\Gamma\left(n_{ij}+\alpha_i+\beta_i\right)}$$

($i=1,\ldots,T$; $j=1,\ldots,J_i$), where $\Gamma(\cdot)$ is the gamma function (Johnson and Kotz, 1969, §1.3). Under the reparameterization $\mu_i = \alpha_i/(\alpha_i+\beta_i)$, $\varphi_i = 1/(\alpha_i+\beta_i)$, the mean of Z_{ij} is $E(Z_{ij} \mid n_{ij}) = \mu_i$, and the variance is $var(Z_{ij} \mid n_{ij}) = n_{ij}^{-1}\mu_i(1-\mu_i)\{1 + (n_{ij}-1)\varphi_i/(1+\varphi_i)\}$. In addition, the model now allows for an *intralitter* correlation parameter (Kupper et al., 1986): $\rho_i = Corr(Y_{ijk}, Y_{ijk'}) = \varphi_i/(1 + \varphi_i)$.

Application of the beta-binomial model to developmental toxicity data was first suggested by Williams (1975). Haseman and Kupper (1979) and Kupper et al. (1986) provide useful details on estimation of the μ_i and φ_i. Confidence intervals or tests of hypotheses among the μ_i or ρ_i are also available (Crowder, 1978; Crowder, 1979).

The extra parameterization inherent in modeling φ_i or ρ_i endows the beta-binomial with enhanced flexibility, which often results in better fits to teratogenicity data than, say, binomial or Poisson sampling models for Y_{ij} (Shirley and Hickling, 1981). Indeed, the beta-binomial has been shown to fit teratogenicity data better than other complex generalized binomial models (Paul, 1982), and tests of hypotheses based on the beta-binomial model can exhibit good power to detect departures from the null effect (Pack, 1986). We note, however, that this model adequacy is not ubiquitous: Haseman and Soares (1976) report difficulty in fitting the beta-binomial to their dominant lethal data.

For those teratogenicity studies where the beta-binomial model is considered appropriate, the effects of additional covariates or other explanatory variables may be examined via logistic regression models (Williams, 1982). For example, if a quantitative dose variable, d_i, is associated with each treatment level i ($i=1,\ldots,T$) and d_i is employed as a single explanatory variable, a log-linear logistic link between μ_i and d_i is

$$\mu_i = 1/(1 + exp\{-\gamma_0 - \gamma_1 ln(d_i)\}) .$$

Corresponding significance tests of $H_0{:}\gamma_1=0$ can suggest existence of or lack of a significant dose-response (Kupper et al., 1986).

The Rai-van Ryzin model

A recent parametric construction for teratogenicity data that attempts to model maternal toxicity is the Rai-van Ryzin (RVR) model (Rai and van Ryzin, 1985). It relates maternal effects to fetal effects by setting the probability of female toxic response at dose d of a chemical stimulus to

$$\lambda(d) \equiv \Pr\{\text{toxicity at d}\} = 1 - exp\{-\alpha - \beta d\} .$$

Then, the probability of observing an affected fetus among the n_{ij} fetuses from the jth litter exposed to dose d_i is modeled as $p_{ij} = \lambda(d_i) exp\{-n_{ij}(\theta_1 + \theta_2 d_i)\}$. A surprisingly similar model has been successfully fit to data from the well-known Ames/*Salmonella* mutagenicity assay (Margolin et al., 1989).

Conditional on the n_{ij}, the Y_{ij} are assumed to be binomially distributed with parameters n_{ij} and p_{ij}. Any extra-binomial variability in Y_{ij} is assumed accounted-for in the RVR model by inclusion of covariates into the exponential portion multiplying n_{ij} in p_{ij}. For example, the above expression for p_{ij} employs dose, d_i, as a covariate.

One additional feature of the RVR model is the inclusion in the model of a discrete probability distribution for the n_{ij}. RVR (1985) suggest a Poisson model for n_{ij}. Based on these various components, estimates of the parameters may be calculated (Rai and van Ryzin, 1985), and hypothesis tests are also available. For instance, H_0:θ_2=0 tests for a significant dose-response.

Although the RVR approach has been applied successfully in certain applications (Faustman et al., 1989), Williams (1987) notes that the model adjusts for extra-binomial variability by assuming such variability is wholly attributable to the influence of (changing) litter sizes (possibly modified by any covariables). He indicates that this assumption may be too restrictive. Carr and Portier (1990) also identify this possibility. They show that simply controlling litter size is not sufficient to account for the extra-binomial variability they observe in a large base of teratogenicity data. Clearly, further refinement of the RVR approach is in order before it can be recommended for use.

Quasi-likelihood for (generalized) linear modeling

One recent development in statistical theory that has application to per-litter analyses is the construction of schemes that relax specific distributional assumptions for the observations. Only limited assumptions on the mean and variance are required, which are employed to construct quasi-likelihood estimating equations for the mean parameters (McCullagh and Nelder, 1983, §8).

In order to accommodate the linear model, let Z_ℓ indicate the ℓth per-litter observed proportion (ℓ=1,...,L; $L=\sum_1^T J_i$). Associated with each Z_ℓ is a litter size n_ℓ and a set of M≥1 recorded predictor variables $[x_{\ell 1}\ x_{\ell 2} \cdots x_{\ell M}]'$. The mean response, μ_ℓ, for each Z_ℓ is linked to a linear predictor, $\eta_\ell = \sum_{m=1}^M \beta_m x_{\ell m}$ via some function $\eta_\ell = g(\mu_\ell)$. For example, Williams (1982) presents quasi-likelihood analyses based on a logistic link: $g(\mu) = ln\{\mu/(1-\mu)\}$. His procedure can be regarded as a generalization of a weighted least squares approach (Cochran, 1943; Kleinman, 1973). From this, estimators, $\hat{\beta}_m$, of the β_m are assembled, along with standard errors and correlations among the $\hat{\beta}_m$.

One consequence of the quasi-likelihood model is the incorporation of overdispersion into the required moment assumptions. Suppose the variance of Z_ℓ takes the form $\text{var}(Z_\ell \mid n_\ell) = \mu_\ell(1-\mu_\ell)\{1 + \rho(n_\ell-1)/n_\ell\}/n_\ell$, where ρ is some dispersion parameter (Moore, 1986; Williams, 1982). This form is similar to the beta-binomial variance encountered above, except that no specific distributional characterization (beta-binomial or otherwise) is placed on the sampling distribution of the Y_{ij}. Moore (1986) suggests a generalization of this variance model to allow for other forms of overdispersion. He also provides estimates of the variances and correlations among these parameter estimates, for use in constructing confidence intervals or significance tests.

Quasi-likelihood for longitudinal outcomes

Liang and Zeger (1986) present a quasi-likelihood approach for linear models that can be formulated to model intralitter correlation directly, rather than with a dispersion parameter. Their approach is more flexible; it allows for modelling of any fetus-specific (rather than simply litter-specific) explanatory variables. One simply views the ℓth female's n_ℓ fetal responses as a single longitudinal response vector for that female. The intralitter correlation is then the per-female longitudinal correlation. Additional predictor variables (such as dose) are incorporated via a generalized linear model, as above. Confidence intervals and significance tests are also available. This modeling approach has been extended by Zeger et al. (1988), and Prentice (1988).

Some simplifications for analyzing multiple outcomes under a longitudinal approach have been noted by Lefkopoulou et al. (1989), and a further computational extension involving bootstrapping has also appeared (Moulton and Zeger, 1989). In a comparison of various quasi-likelihood approaches to teratogenicity data analysis, however, Carr (1989) found no single method to be uniformly superior under beta-binomial sampling when no fetus-specific variates were considered.

Extensions: Risk estimation

There is, of course, the additional problem of *extrapolating* results from a developmental toxicity assay in rodents to potential toxic effects in humans (Gaylor, 1989). This issue has clear importance and impact (Hogan and Hoel, 1989; Johnson, 1988; Khera et al., 1989, Ch. 9). Specific quantitative concerns involve estimation of so-called "acceptable" levels for humans exposures, based on observed rodent teratogenic dose-responses (Chen and Kodell, 1989; Kaplan et al., 1987; Kimmel and Gaylor, 1988). In this instance, parametric models are more centrally involved, since extrapolations over the low-dose regions are easier to calculate when, say, a beta-binomial model with a log-linear logistic link is assumed to hold (Kupper et al., 1986). Nonetheless, the choice of parametric model must be made carefully, so as not to invalidate or misinterpret the inferences attained from the statistical analysis. As a minimally-parametric alternative for such risk estimation settings, Carr (1989) notes that the bootstrap approach can allow for inferences on low-exposure characteristics without necessarily invoking heavily-parameterized models.

Acknowledgements

Our thanks to Drs. D.D. Boos, G.J. Carr, L. Edler, B.C. Gladen, L. Hothorn, C.J. Portier, M.D. Shelby, and P. Williams for helpful recommendations in the preparation of this material.

References

Aeschbacher HU, Vuataz L, Sotek J, Stalder R (1977) Use of the beta-binomial distribution in dominant-lethal testing for "weak mutagenic activity". Mutat. Res. 44:369-390.

Anscombe FJ (1948) The transformation of Poisson, binomial and negative binomial data. Biometrika 35:246-254.

Becker BA (1974) The statistics of teratology. Teratol. 9:261-261.

Brier SS, Zacks S, Marlow WH (1986) An application of empirical Bayes techniques to the simultaneous estimation of many probabilities. Naval Res. Logis. Q. 33:77-90.

Carr GJ (1989) Dose-response models in quantal response teratology. Ph.D. thesis, University of North Carolina, Chapel Hill.

Carr GJ, Portier CJ (1990) An evaluation of the Rai and van Ryzin dose-response model in teratology. Risk Anal. (to appear).

Chen JJ, Kodell RL (1989) Quantitative risk assessment for teratological effects. J. Amer. Statist. Assoc. 84:966-971.

Cochran WG (1943) Analysis of variance for percentages based on unequal numbers. J. Amer. Statist. Assoc. 38:287-301.

Crowder MJ (1978) Beta-binomial ANOVA for proportions. Appl. Statist. 27:34-37.

Crowder MJ (1979) Inference about the intraclass correlation coefficient in the beta-binomial ANOVA for proportions. J. Roy. Statist. Soc., ser. B 41:230-234.

Efron B (1982) The Jackknife, the Bootstrap and Other Resampling Plans. Society for Industrial and Applied Mathematics, Philadelphia.

Ehling UH, Machemer L, Buselmaier W, Dycka J, Frohberg H, Kratochvilova J, Lang R, Lorke D, Mueller D, Peh J, Roehrborn G, Roll R, Schulze-Schencking M, Weimann H (1978) Standard protocol for the dominant lethal test on male mice set up by the work group "Dominant lethal mutations of the ad hoc committee chemogenetics". Arch. Toxicol. 39:173-185.

Epstein SS, Arnold E, Andrea J, Bass W, Bishop Y (1972) Detection of chemical mutagens by the dominant lethal assay in the mouse. Toxicol. Appl. Pharmacol. 23:288-325.

Faustman EM, Wellington DG, Smith GP, Kimmel CA (1989) Characterization of a developmental toxicity dose-response model. Env. Health Persp. 79:229-241.

Frangos CC, Stone M (1984) On jackknife, cross-validatory and classical methods of estimating a proportion with batches of different sizes. Biometrika 71:361-366.

Gad S, Weil CS (1986) Statistics and Experimental Design for Toxicologists. Telford Press, Caldwell, NJ.

Gaylor DW (1989) Quantitative risk analysis for quantal reproductive and developmental effects. Env. Health Persp. 79:243-246.

Gladen B (1979) The use of the jackknife to estimate proportions from toxicological data in the presence of litter effects. J. Amer. Statist. Assoc. 74:278-282.

Haseman JK, Hoel DG (1974) Tables of Gehan's generalized Wilcoxon test with fixed point censoring. J. Statist. Comput. Simul. 3:117-135.

Haseman JK, Hogan MD (1975) Selection of the experimental unit in teratology studies. Teratol. 12:165-172.

Haseman JK, Kupper LL (1979) Analysis of dichotomous response data from certain toxicological experiments. Biometrics 35:281-293.

Haseman JK, Soares ER (1976) The distribution of fetal death in control mice and its implications on statistical tests for dominant lethal effects. Mutat. Res. 41:277-288.

Healy MJR (1972) Animal litters as experimental units. Appl. Statist. 21:155-159.

Hogan MD, Hoel DG (1989) Extrapolation to man (2nd ed.). In: Hayes AW (ed) Principles and Methods of Toxicology, Raven Press, New York, 879-892.

James DA, Smith DM (1982) Analysis of results from a collaborative study of the dominant lethal assay. Mutat. Res. 97:303-314.

Johnson EM (1988) Cross-species extrapolations and the biological basis for safety factor determinations in developmental toxicology. Reg. Toxicol. Pharmacol. 8:22-36.

Johnson NL, Kotz S (1969) Distributions in Statistics: Discrete Distributions. Houghton-Mifflin, Boston.

Johnson NL, Kotz S (1970) Continuous Univariate Distributions — 2. Wiley, New York.

Kalter H (1974) The choice of the number of sampling units in teratology. Teratol. 9:257-258.

Kaplan N, Hoel DG, Portier CJ, Hogan MD (1987) An evaluation of the safety factor approach in risk assessment. In: McLachlan JA, Pratt RM, Markert CL (eds) Developmental Toxicity: Mechanisms and Risks, vol 26, Cold Spring Harbor Laboratory, Cold Spring Harbor, NY, 335-344.

Khera KS, Grice HC, Clegg DJ (eds) (1989) Current issues in Toxicology: Interpretation and Extrapolation of Reproductive Data to Establish Human Safety Standards. Springer-Verlag, New York.

Kimmel CA, Gaylor DW (1988) Issues in qualitative and quantitative risk analysis for developmental toxicology. Risk Anal. 8:15-20.

Kleinman JC (1973) Proportions with extraneous variance: Single and independent samples. J. Amer. Statist. Assoc. 68:46-54.

Kupper LL, Portier CJ, Hogan MD, Yamamoto E (1986) The impact of litter effects on dose-response modeling in teratology. Biometrics 42:85-98.

Lamb JCI, Moore JA, Marks TA, Haseman JK (1981) Development and viability of offspring of male mice treated with chlorinated phenoxy acids and 2,3,7,8-tetrachlorodibenzo-p-dioxin. J. Toxicol. Env. Health 8:835-844.

Lefkopoulou M, Moore D, Ryan L (1989) The analysis of multiple correlated binary outcomes: Applications to rodent teratology experiments. J. Amer. Statist. Assoc. 84:810-815.

Lehmann EL (1975) Nonparametrics: Statistical Methods Based on Ranks. Holden-Day, San Francisco.

Liang KY, Zeger SL (1986) Longitudinal data analysis using generalized linear models. Biometrika 73:13-22.

Lin FO, Haseman JK (1976) A modified Jonckheere test against ordered alternatives when ties are present at a single extreme value. Biom. Z. 18:623-631.

Manson JM, Kang YJ (1989) Test methods for assessing female reproductive and developmental toxicology (2nd ed.). In: Hayes AW (ed) Principles and Methods of Toxicology, Raven Press, New York, 311-360.

Mantel N (1979) Ridit analysis and related ranking procedures — Use at your own risk. Amer. J. Epidemiol. 109:25-29.

Margolin BH, Kim BS, Risko KJ (1989) The Ames *salmonella*/microsome mutagenicity assay: Issues of inference and validation. J. Amer. Statist. Assoc. 84:651-661.

McCullagh P, Nelder JA (1983) Generalized Linear Models. Chapman and Hall, London.

McLachlan JA, Pratt RM, Markert CL (eds) (1987) Developmental Toxicity: Mechanisms and Risks. Cold Spring Harbor Laboratory, Cold Spring Harbor, NY.

Miller RG (1981) Simultaneous Statistical Inference (2nd ed.). Springer-Verlag, New York.

Moore DF (1986) Asymptotic properties of moment estimators for overdispersed counts and proportions. Biometrika 73:583-588.

Moulton LH, Zeger SL (1989) Analyzing repeated measures on generalized linear models via the bootstrap. Biometrics 45:381-394.

Pack SE (1986) Hypothesis testing with overdispersion. Biometrics 42:967-972.

Pasternack BS, Shore RE (1982) Analysis of dichotomous response data from toxicological experiments involving stable laboratory mouse populations. Biometrics 38:1057-1067.

Paul SR (1982) Analysis of proportions of affected foetuses in teratological experiments. Biometrics 38:361-370.

Paul SR, Mantel N (1989) Model-free analysis of litter-depletion data. The Statist. 38:121-125.

Prentice RL (1988) Correlated binary regression with covariates specific to each binary observation. Biometrics 44:1033-1048.

Quenouille MH (1949) Approximate tests of correlation in time series. J. Roy. Statist. Soc., ser. B 11:68-84.

Rai K, van Ryzin J (1985) A dose-response model for teratological experiments involving quantal response. Biometrics 41:1-9.

Shirley EAC, Hickling R (1981) An evaluation of some statistical methods for analyzing numbers of abnormalities found amongst litters in teratology studies. Biometrics 37:819-829.

Simpson DG, Margolin BH (1986) Recursive nonparametric testing for dose-response relationships subject to downturns at high doses. Biometrika 73:589-596.

Vuataz L, Sotek J (1978) Use of the beta-binomial distribution in dominant-lethal testing for "weak mutagenic activity". Mutat. Res. 52:211-230.

Weil CS (1970) Selection of the valid number of sampling units and a consideration of their combination in toxicological studies involving reproduction, teratogenesis, or carcinogenesis. Fd. Cosm. Toxicol. 8:177-182.

Williams DA (1975) The analysis of binary responses from toxicological experiments involving reproduction and teratogenicity. Biometrics 31:949-952.

Williams DA (1982) Extra-binomial variation in logistic linear models. Appl. Statist. 31:144-148.

Williams DA (1987) Dose-response models for teratological experiments. Biometrics 43:1013-1016.

Zeger SL, Liang K-Y, Albert PS (1988) Models for longitudinal data: A generalized estimating equation approach. Biometrics 44:1049-1060.

Biometrical Analysis of Strain Differences and Litter Effects.

A Case Study

Reinhard Meister[1], Ibrahim Chahoud, Maike Jürgens, Frank Iversen, Gerd Bochert
[1]Technische Fachhochschule Berlin, FB 2 Luxemburger Straße 10, D1000 Berlin 65
Freie Universität Berlin, Institut für Toxikologie und Embryopharmakologie

1. Introduction

There are different ways of dealing with biological problems in order to find an appropriate biometrical analysis. These approaches correspond to different objectives:

- to increase efficiency
  variance reduction, power optimization, etc.

- to decrease bias
  adjusting for covariables, including systematic factors, etc.

We will focus on the second objective in this paper, as we want to emphasize the importance of a proper understanding of the biological problem examining *reproductive toxicity.* The first objective is very important for the development of theoretical statistics, but not always of practical relevance. The bias induced by incorrect understanding of the biological problem, however, can be much larger than any possible gain in efficiency.

In animal studies on reproductive toxicity, the parents are assigned at random to different treatment groups and the effects of the treatments are evaluated on the offspring — e.g. embryos, fetuses or pups. Most papers – i.e. Kleinman (1973), Kupper and Haseman (1978), Haseman and Kupper (1979), Gladen (1979), Rai and Van Ryzin (1985), Kupper et al. (1986), Williams (1975, 82, 87) – dealing with the biometrical analysis of this type of experiments solely discuss the issue of litter effects, but there are a lot of other topics important for a proper understanding of events observed in prenatal toxicity testing – Neubert et al. (1987). We will address some of these points in the next paragraph.

2. Endpoints and predictors of prenatal toxicity

The nature of a problem can be determined by the characterization of possible response variables and factors which may have some influence on the results. Only through a continuous discussion between the statistician and the applied researchers can an appropriate understanding of the biological background necessary for an adequate statistical model be achieved.
For the typical experimental setup in prenatal toxicity testing, we consider the following responses — called endpoints — and factors as important:

- endpoints:
  mortality, structural and functional anomalies, transplacental carcinogenicity
- factors:
  - given by experimental design
    species, phase, substance, dose
  - confounders
    litters, sex, maternal toxicity, mortality

The endpoints are mostly given as dichotomous data, called *quantal response*. Among the possible effects mortality is a very severe but not very specific response with respect to risk extrapolation for man. The elucidation of the induction of gross-structural abnormalities is the subject of what is called *teratology*, but the field of interest for assessing toxic effects during the reproductive cycle is much broader and includes effects which can only be detected in the young or grown-up offspring of treated parents. Such effects are e.g. cerebral anomalies or transplacental carcinogenicity.

The factors not under the control of the experimenter — called confounders — can make a proper analysis of the results difficult or even impossible. We will explain this effect for the case of increased mortality, an endpoint which may raise problems for the estimation of the probability of other anomalies under study. As can be seen in our list, mortality appears twice, as endpoint as well as confounder. Therefore, the evaluation is rather difficult.

Ignoring the litter structure of our experimental groups, the results for a given treatment group may be denoted by n, s, r, where n is the number of *implantations*, s is the number of *surviving* fetuses and r is the number of *responders* – living fetuses showing a certain abnormality (e.g. cleft palate). We further define some events of interest: A will denote the event that an *abnormality* has been induced, M will denote *mortality* which is fetal death and by S we will indicate the *survival* of a fetus. As mortality and survival are complementary events we have $M^C = S$. From the observed values for n, s, r we derive estimators as follows: we estimate $P(A|S)$, the conditional probability for an anomaly of a living fetus by r/s and the unconditional probability for fetal death by $(n-s)/n$. We get the theoretical unconditional probability for an abnormality easily as

$$P(A) = P(A|S)P(S) + P(A|M)P(M)$$

but in practice we cannot decide whether a fetus has carried the abnormality if it died during pregnancy. Therefore, we cannot find estimators for $P(A|M)$ and, consequently,

$P(M)$	$P(A\|S)$					
	0.1		**0.25**		**0.5**	
0.1	0.09	0.19	0.225	0.325	0.45	0.55
0.25	0.075	0.325	0.1875	0.4375	0.375	0.625
0.5	0.05	0.55	0.125	0.625	0.25	0.75

Table 1: Possible true response probabilities $P(A)$ for different rates of mortality $P(M)$ and abnormalities among the living $P(A|S)$. The lower values correspond to the assumption $P(A|M) = 0$, the higher to $P(A|M) = 1$.

for $P(A)$. Independence between mortality and the induction of an anomaly would allow to use r/s as an unbiased estimator. Otherwise, the proportion of affected among the living fetuses will yield a biased estimator. To illustrate the possible bias we calculated the values of table 1 assuming $P(A|M) = 0$ and $P(A|M) = 1$.

The effect of underestimating the true probability of an abnormality can be so strong, that decreasing rates of abnormalities can be observed if mortality increases substantially.

As there is no mathematical way to circumvent this effect, the experimental setup has to be changed if we want to avoid it.

One possible reason for increased mortality is the long-term treatment of animals due to regulatory demands. Long-term treatment during a substantial part of the whole reproductive cycle is demanded in order to have the chance to observe the induction of abnormalities at all possible critical periods of development. The price of this approach can be biased estimates of malformation rates.

If the susceptible period for the induction of a given effect is known, treatment at a single time during pregnancy can yield much more specific information, avoiding the described drawback of long-term treatment. The proper choice and adjustment of time of treatment will be discussed in the next part.

3. Removing strain differences – An example

Time specific effects are often observed in teratology. This seems to be reasonable since certain effects can only be induced during a short time intervall where an organ is in the critical stage of development. If treatment takes place before or some time after this critical stage, a low or no effect will be observed. Difficulties arise if a short-term treatment at a given time during pregnancy yields different response rates in different groups of animals. Even between different strains of the same species such differences are known to exist. Again, a bias can be generated if results of a certain strain are used to make a risk assessment for man.

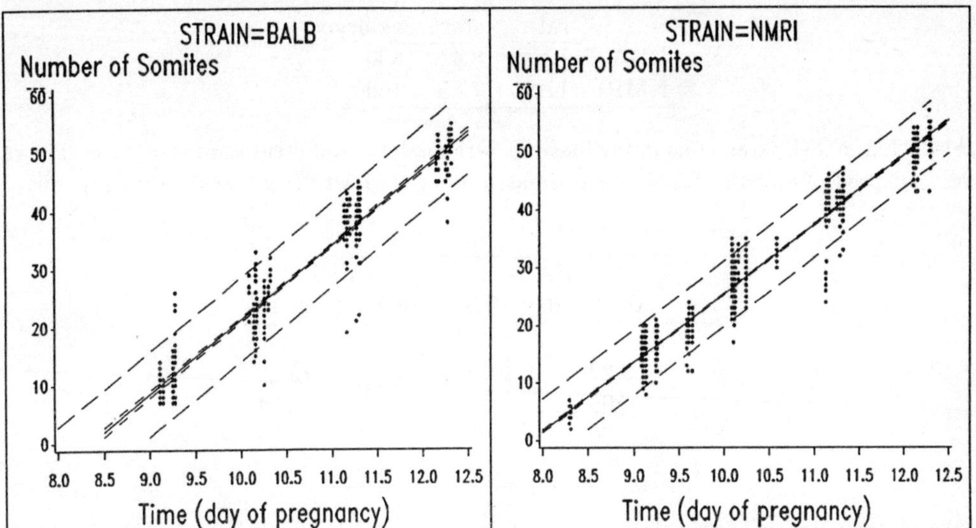

Figure 1: Somite growth for two strains of mice. The linear regression curves including 95% confidence intervals for the individual and the mean values are given. Possible litter-effects are ignored.

For all mammalian species there are similar stages of embryonic development, but these stages are reached within different time schedules. In rodents a strong relationship between the developmental stage and the number of somites has been proven. These facts are used to demonstrate how strain differences can be explained and almost be removed, if an adjustment of time is made with respect to the developmental stage of the animals. In our laboratory we have extensive experience with studies on the teratogenic potency of methyl-nitroso-urea (MNU) in rodents. MNU is an alkylating agent with an extremely short half-life. It can be used as a model-compound to demonstrate the time specificity of an effect – Platzek et al. (1989). On the other hand, we have sampled data on the somite numbers of embryos during different times of pregnancy. We will use some of these data to illustrate our proposal for time adjustment of treatments to the developmental stage. A comprehensive description of these experiments can be found in Chahoud et al. (1991)..

We make the following assumptions:

- The developmental stage determines the susceptibility against a given treatment.
- The number of somites characterizes the stage of development.
- The growth curve for the somite numbers can be approximated sufficiently by a straight line.

With this assumptions it is possible to choose appropriate treatment times for different strains, such that treatment is given at a similar stage of development.

We analysed the somite growth for two strains of mice – the DBA and the NMRI strain. We see from figure 1 that our assumption on the functional form of the growth-curve is reasonable.

	rate	start	embryos
DBA	12.25	8.4	600
NMRI	11.95	7.85	1500

Table 2: Estimated parameters in the linear growth model for different strains of mice. The rate gives the speed of growth, start is the estimated onset of growth (e.g. $\mathrm{E}(som(start)) = 0$).

	DBA		NMRI	
	day 10	day 10.5	day 9.5	day 10
$\hat{p}$	0.22	0.65	0.10	0.89
n	109	27	220	134
l	30	5	22	10
DI	2.3	5.2	3.2	2.6

Table 3: Induction of cleft palates by treatment with MNU (5 mg/kg ip). The estimated response rate $\hat{p}$, the total number of living fetuses n, the number of litters l and the ratio $DI = \hat{\sigma}^2_{\hat{p}}/(n^{-1}\hat{p}(1-\hat{p}))$ of the estimated variance – Gladen (1979) – to that expected under the binomial model are given for different times of treatment.

From the parameter estimates given in table 2 we deduce that somite growth procedes with a similar rate in these two strains – about one somite every two hours – but the DBA strain starts with approximately half a day delay.

If we consider a treatment on day 10 of pregnancy we expect a somite number of $(10 - 7.85) \times 11.95 = 24.6$ somites for the NMRI strain. This stage will be reached by the DBA strain after $24.6/12.25 + 8.4 = 10.4$ days of pregnancy. The good agreement of our prediction with the experimental results can be found in table 3.

4. Sources of extra binomial variation for quantal response data in prenatal toxicology

All fetuses of a litter grow in the same uterus. Therefore, we have no reason to expect them to react independently to a treatment of the mother. This problem is known as *litter effect* in prenatal toxicology. Litter effects are observed for continuous as well as for quantal response data. We give a brief overview how these effects can be modeled and described.

Notations for a group of litters: Let us denote by y_{ij} the observation for the j–th fetus of the i–th litter, $i = 1, \cdots, l; l$ is the number of litters ; $j = 1, \cdots, n_i; n_i$ is the size of the i–th litter. We use $n = \sum_i n_i$ for the total number of fetuses and for quantal response data we use z instead of y. The general null hypothesis is H_0: no litter effect.

We summarize the different approaches for the incorporation of litter effects by the following list. We will not discuss details of these aproaches and refer to the given literature.

Continuous variables

- Variance components — Healy (1972)
  $y_{ij} = \mu + w_i + e_{ij}, Ew_i = Ee_{ij} = 0 \; \{w_i, e_{ij}\}; \{e_{ij}\}; \{w_i\}$ uncorrelated
  with $Vw_i = \sigma_w^2, Ve_{ij} = \sigma^2$
  $H_0: \quad \sigma_w^2 = 0$

- Covariances
  $y_{ij} = \mu + e_{ij}, Cov(e_{i_1 j_1}, e_{i_2 j_2}) = \delta_{i_1 i_2} \rho \sigma^2$
  $H_0: \quad \rho = 0$

- Covariables
  $y_{ij} = \mu + x_i^T \beta + e_{ij}$
  $H_0: \quad \beta = 0$

Estimation and tests: Linear Models.

Quantal response

H_0: z_{ij} iid B$(1,p)$ is used for all alternativ approaches

- alternative distributions — Williams (1975), Kupper & Haseman, Altham (1978)
- alternative variance formulae — Kleinmann (1973), Williams (1982), Gladen (1979)
- concept of correlated tolerances

The drawback of the approaches for quantal response data compared to the case of continuous data is the lack of an easy biological interpretation for the deviations from the null hypothesis. Stating that there is a discrete probability distribution showing a variance different from the binomial has no direct biological meaning. On the other hand, it is the usual interpretation of block-effects which makes the variance component models or the incorporation of correlations so attractive for the biologist. We, therefore, recommend that a more interpretable approach should be developed. If we remember that all quantal response models can be deduced from assumptions on the underlying tolerance distribution we have the possibility to state deviations from the no-litter-effect hypothesis in terms of the continuous variables models.

For our example we have tried to associate the observed litter effects on the somite numbers during different stages (see figure 2) with the observed overdispersion of the estimated response rate, but we could not find any obvious relationship. If we can find out how a given tolerance distribution and assumptions on the error structure will influence the variance of the estimated response probability, we will be able to get the desired interpretation.

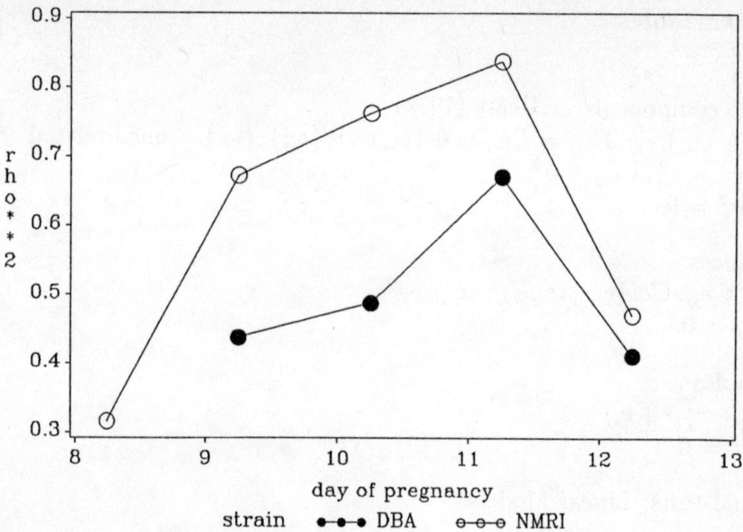

Figure 2: Intralitter correlations during different times of pregnancy. The correlations $\hat{\rho}^2 := \hat{\sigma}_l^2/(\hat{\sigma}_l^2 + \hat{\sigma}_e^2)$ are derived from estimates of the variance components ($\hat{\sigma}_l^2$ – litters; $\hat{\sigma}_e^2$ – error) for the somite numbers. The results are given for DBA and NMRI mice.

depends on the correlation between the individual tolerances y_{ij}. For a fixed response rate, the overdispersion seems to show a linear dependence on ρ^2.

5. Discussion

Animal studies on the risk assessment of toxic effects for man can be biased if the selection of different strains is critical. We have demonstrated that strain differences in prenatal toxicity testing can be explained and partially removed if information on developmental biology is incorporated into the biometrical analysis. There are confounders like mortality where bias can only be avoided by an appropriate study design.

There are special questions in teratology – like the problem litter effect for quantal response data – where uptill now the biological meaning of statistical findings is not obvious. The proposed concept of correlated tolerances may be a way to improve the interpretability of litter-effect models.

6. Acknowledgement

Parts of this work were supported by grants from the Deutsche Forschungsgemeinschaft given to the Sonderforschungsbereich 174 — Risikoabschätzung von vorgeburtlichen Schädigungen.

7. References

Altham PME (1978) Two generalizations of the binomial distribution. Applied Statistics 27: 162-167

Chahoud I, Bochert G, Jürgens M, Neubert D (1991) Embryonic development and strain differences. Arch Toxicol (in prep)

Gladen B (1979) The use of the Jackknife to estimate proportions from toxicological data in the presence of litter effects. JASA 74: 278-283

Haseman JK, Kupper LL (1979) Analysis of dichotomous response data from certain toxicological experiments. Biometrics 35: 281-293.

Healy MJR (1972) Animal litters as experimental units. Applied Statistics 21: 155-159

Kleinmann JC (1973) Proportions with extranous variance: single and independent samples JASA 68: 46-54

Kupper LL, Haseman JK (1978) The use of a correlated binomial model for the analysis of certain toxicological experiments. Biometrics 34: 69-76

Kupper LL, Hogan MD, Portier C, Yamamoto E (1986) The impact of litter effects on dose-response modeling in teratology. Biometrics 42: 85-98

Neubert D, Chahoud I, Platzek T, Meister R (1987) Principles and problems in assessing prenatal toxicity. Arch Toxicol 60: 238-245

Platzek T, Bochert G, Pauli B, Meister R, Neubert D (1988) Embryotoxicity induced by alkylating agents: 5. Dose-response relationships of teratogenic effects of methyl-nitroso urea in mice. Arch Toxicol 62:411-423

Rai K, Van Ryzin J (1985) A dose-response model for teratological experiments involving quantal response. Biometrics 41: 1-9

Williams DA (1975) The analysis of binary response from toxicological experiments involving reproduction and teratogenicity. Biometrics 31: 949-952

Williams DA (1982) Extra-binomial variation in logistic linear models. Applied statistics 31: 144-148

Williams DA (1987) Dose response models for teratological experiments. Biometrics 43: 1013-1016

Statistical Evaluation of Offspring Parameters in Embryotoxicity Studies

G. Rosenkranz, R. Uhl
Hoechst AG
Pharma Forschung Informatik
W-6230 Frankfurt am Main 80, FRG

1 Introduction

Embryotoxicity studies are used to assess the extent to which a substance may have harmful effects on the offspring of treated animals. Among other things the size or weight of the offspring or the placental weights have to be assessed for treatment induced changes. These assessments are complicated by the fact that treatment only affects the foetuses indirectly via the mother animal in addition to which the individual foetus cannot be maintained under controllable conditions. It can, therefore, be supposed that animals from different dams are subject to different influences during intrauterine development, which are not primarily induced by treatment. The statistical evaluation of the study must take this "litter effect" into account.

The two extreme points of view that can be taken in the evaluation of fetal data and their effects on the statistical analysis are explained in the following. If the view is taken that the fact that a foetus belongs to a certain litter does not influence the analysis, then assigning the individual foetuses to specific litters is irrelevant. The best indicator of the mean value for a parameter, e.g. mean body weight, would be the arithmetic mean calculated from all individual values or, the *weighted* arithmetic mean of litter means, the litter sizes being the weighting factors. The other extreme is the view that differences only exist within litters and not between litters. In this case, a good indicator for the mean value for a parameter would be the *unweighted* mean of the litter mean values. In reality, however, there is a mixture of both extremes. This shows that a statistical analysis which is based on unweighted litter means or litter means weighted by the litter size offers no solution to the problem.

In the present paper we review some statistical methods which are possible approaches for the analysis of continuous fetal data. Each method presupposes that the data can be modeled by a mixed hierarchical linear model. In this model, the litter effect is described by a nested random factor and dosage by a fixed factor. According to Searle (1987) such a model can be formulated as follows:

$$\mathsf{Y} = \mathsf{X}_0\beta_0 + \mathsf{X}_1\beta_1 + \mathsf{e}$$

where

- Y is an n-vector of observations (e.g., fetal weight),
- X_0 and X_1 are known design matrices,
- β_0 is the vector of the fixed effect (i.e., group or dosage),
- β_1 is the vector of the random effect (i.e., litter),
- e is an n-vector of random errors.

Furthermore we suppose that (I denotes the identity matrix)

- e is normally distributed with mean zero and covariance matrix $\sigma_0^2\mathsf{I}$,
- β_1 is normally distributed with mean zero and covariance matrix $\sigma_1^2\mathsf{I}$,
- β_1 and e are independent.

If E denotes expectation and V variance then

$$\begin{aligned} \mathsf{E}[\mathsf{Y}] &= \mathsf{X}_0\beta_0 \\ \mathsf{V}[\mathsf{Y}] &= \mathsf{X}_1\mathsf{X}_1'\sigma_1^2 + \sigma_0^2\mathsf{I} \end{aligned}$$

holds. (X' denotes the transpose of X.)

In the main part of the paper we discuss two methods based on least squares and two based on the likelihood principle. For this discussion we assume that an experiment with g groups shall be analyzed. Furthermore n_i denotes the number of dams in group i, and n_{ij} the number of fetuses of dam j in group i. The total number of observations n is then given by $\sum_{i=1}^{g}\sum_{j=1}^{n_i} n_{ij}$. In our case, β_0 and β_1 are given by

$$\begin{aligned} \beta_0 &= (\mu, \alpha_1, \ldots, \alpha_g) \\ \beta_1 &= (\gamma_{11}, \ldots, \gamma_{gn_g}). \end{aligned}$$

Note that μ denotes grand mean, the α's correspond to the group effect and the γ's to the random hierarchical litter effect. Our primary interest is to obtain a test for no group effect, i.e. we want to test the hypotheses

$$H_i : \alpha_i - \alpha_1 = 0, \quad i = 2, \ldots, g.$$

σ_0^2 measures the variability *between* litters and σ_1^2 the variability *within* litters. Hence for a litter with k fetuses, the variance of the litter mean of Y is given by $\sigma_0^2 + \sigma_1^2/k$. If σ_0^2 or σ_1^2 is set to zero, the two aforementioned extreme situations are obtained.

The main problem of the statistical analysis of such a model stems from the fact that the study design is in general highly unbalanced, because the number of fetuses per dam varies strongly. Unbalance is the reason why many proposals fail to provide a valid solution for the statistical analysis of offspring data.

2 Least-squares based Methods

2.1 Healy's Approach

One of the first papers which dealt with the analysis of continuous offspring parameters was Healy (1972). In this article, an extension of the analysis of variance method is described to estimate the variance components σ_0^2 and σ_1^2. With these estimators weighted litter means are calculated and the weighted means of the treated groups are compared to those of the control by means of a t-test. If MSL denotes the mean sum of squares between litters and MSE denotes the mean sum of squares within litters we obtain

$$\begin{aligned} \mathsf{E}[\mathrm{MSE}] &= \sigma_0^2, \\ \mathsf{E}[\mathrm{MSL}] &= k\sigma_1^2 + \sigma_0^2, \end{aligned}$$

with

$$k = \frac{n - \sum_{i,j}(n_{ij}^2/\sum_j n_{ij})}{\sum_i (n_i - 1)}.$$

(Gower, 1962; Gates and Chiue, 1962). Hence

$$\begin{aligned} s_0^2 &= \mathrm{MSE} \\ s_1^2 &= (\mathrm{MSL} - \mathrm{MSE})/k \end{aligned}$$

are unbiased estimates for σ_0^2 and σ_1^2, respectively. The weighted means and sum of squares for the t-test are calculated with $1/(s_0^2 + s_1^2/k)$ as weighting factors.

This approach runs into several difficulties. First of all, it is possible that s_1^2 becomes negative. This is a general disadvantage of the analysis-of-variance approach to estimate variance components even if the design is balanced. However the major drawback is, that the distribution of s_1^2 is completely unknown and especially not χ^2 (see Searle, 1987). Therefore the assumptions necessary to do a t-test are not valid in general, at least for finite samples. As far as we know, even asymptotic results are not established at present.

2.2 Fixed-Effect Approach

The second procedure is termed "fixed-effect approach" because the main idea behind it is to formally treat all effects in the model as if they were fixed. To do this let

$$\mathsf{X} = [\mathsf{X}_0, \mathsf{X}_1], \quad \beta = (\beta_0, \beta_1)$$

be the combined design matrix and the combined parameter vector, respectively. Let

$$\mathsf{b} = (\mathsf{X}'\mathsf{X})^{-}\mathsf{X}'\mathsf{Y}$$

be the usual least squares estimator of β. (X^{-} denotes a generalized inverse of X.) For any linear contrast L, i.e., any linear function such that $\mathsf{L}\beta$ is estimable, let

$$\mathrm{SS}(\mathsf{L}) = (\mathsf{Lb})'[\mathsf{L}(\mathsf{X}'\mathsf{X})^{-}\mathsf{L}']^{-1}\mathsf{Lb}$$

the corresponding sum of squares. For our problem we consider the special contrast L_0^i defined by $\mathsf{L}_0^i\beta = \alpha_i - \alpha_1$ and L_1 defined such that $\mathsf{L}_1\beta = 0$ is equivalent to $\gamma_{ij} = 0$ for each i, j. As already mentioned above, the first contrast belongs to the hypothesis of no group effect, the second to the hypothesis of no litter effect. With

$$Q_L = \mathsf{X}(\mathsf{X}'\mathsf{X})^{-}\mathsf{L}'[\mathsf{L}(\mathsf{X}'\mathsf{X})^{-}\mathsf{L}']^{-1}\mathsf{L}(\mathsf{X}'\mathsf{X})^{-}\mathsf{X}'$$

$Q_0^i = Q_{\mathsf{L}_0^i}$, and $Q_1 = Q_{\mathsf{L}_1}$ we obtain

$$\begin{aligned} \mathrm{E}[\mathrm{SS}(\mathsf{L}_0^i)] &= \beta_0'\mathsf{X}_0'Q_0^i\mathsf{X}_0\beta_0 + \mathrm{tr}(\mathsf{X}_1'Q_0^i\mathsf{X}_1)\sigma_1^2 + \sigma_0^2 \\ \mathrm{E}[\mathrm{SS}(\mathsf{L}_1)] &= \mathrm{tr}(\mathsf{X}_1'Q_1\mathsf{X}_1)\sigma_1^2 + \mathrm{rank}(\mathsf{L}_1)\sigma_0^2. \end{aligned}$$

($\mathrm{tr}(\mathsf{X})$ means the trace of the matrix X.) Hence a test for the hypothesis of no group effect can be based on $\mathrm{SS}(\mathsf{L}_0^i)$ and $\mathrm{SS}(\mathsf{L}_1)$. To do this let

$$\mathrm{MS}(\mathsf{L}) = \mathrm{SS}(\mathsf{L})/\mathrm{rank}(\mathsf{L})$$

$$\rho_i = \frac{\mathrm{tr}(\mathsf{X}_1'Q_0^i\mathsf{X}_1)\mathrm{rank}(\mathsf{L}_1)}{\mathrm{tr}(\mathsf{X}_1'Q_1\mathsf{X}_1)}$$

$$\widetilde{\mathrm{MS}}(\mathsf{L}_0^i, \mathsf{L}_1) = \rho_i\mathrm{MS}(\mathsf{L}_1) + (1-\rho_i)\mathrm{MSE}.$$

Then

$$\mathrm{E}[\widetilde{\mathrm{MS}}(\mathsf{L}_0^i, \mathsf{L}_1)|\mathsf{L}_0^i\beta = 0] = \mathrm{E}[\mathrm{MS}(\mathsf{L}_0^i)|\mathsf{L}_0^i\beta = 0]$$

and therefore

$$F_i = \frac{\mathrm{MS}(\mathsf{L}_0^i)}{\widetilde{\mathrm{MS}}(\mathsf{L}_0^i, \mathsf{L}_1)}$$

provides a test statistic for the hypothesis $L_0^i\beta = 0$. The GLM procedure of SAS (SAS Institute, 1988) compares F_i with the upper α-percentile of an F-distribution with one numerator degree of freedom. The denominator degrees of freedom are approximated using Satterthwaite's formula (Satterthwaite, 1946).

The approach is very elegant because it avoids the estimation of variance components. Nevertheless, as with the approach discussed previously, the mean squares contained in the test statistic F_i are not χ^2-distributed in general. Therefore, the F-test just described is not valid, at least for finite sample sizes.

3 Likelihood based Methods

3.1 Maximum Likelihood Approach

Since least squares based methods fail to provide a solution to our basic problem we turn to methods which rely on the maximum likelihood principle. The likelihood for our experimental setting reads

$$l = -\log(\det(V)) - (Y - X_0\beta_0)'V^{-1}(Y - X_0\beta_0)$$

with $V = V[Y]$. l has to be maximized to obtain an estimator for β_0 and the variance components, which are implicit in V. Estimators $\hat{\sigma}_0^2$ and $\hat{\sigma}_1^2$ are obtained from the equations

$$\begin{pmatrix} \mathrm{tr}(\hat{V}^{-2}) & \mathrm{tr}(\hat{V}^{-2}X_1X_1') \\ \mathrm{tr}(\hat{V}^{-1}X_1X_1'\hat{V}^{-1}) & \mathrm{tr}([\hat{V}^{-1}X_1X_1']^2) \end{pmatrix} \begin{pmatrix} \hat{\sigma}_0^2 \\ \hat{\sigma}_1^2 \end{pmatrix} = \begin{pmatrix} Y'\hat{P}^2Y \\ Y'\hat{P}X_1X_1'\hat{P}Y \end{pmatrix}$$

with

$$P = V^{-1}(I - X_0(X_0'V^{-1}X_0)^{-}X_0'V^{-1})$$

(Searle, 1987). Then

$$\hat{b}_0 = (X_0'\hat{V}^{-1}X_0)^{-}X_0'\hat{V}^{-1}Y \tag{1}$$

is the maximum likelihood estimator of β_0. Under the hypothesis of no group effect

$$N_i = \frac{L_0^i\hat{b}_0}{\sqrt{L_0^{i\prime}(X_0'V^{-1}X_0)^{-}L_0^i}} \tag{2}$$

is asymptotically normally distributed with zero mean and variance unity. Replacing V by its estimator $\hat{V}$ yields an asymptotically valid test.

3.2 Restricted Maximum Likelihood Approach

A variant of maximum likelihood estimation in the mixed model is restricted maximum likelihood. The idea is to maximize only that part of the likelihood which is invariant to the fixed effects. If

$$\mathsf{M} = \mathsf{I} - \mathsf{X}_0(\mathsf{X}_0'\mathsf{X}_0)^{-}\mathsf{X}_0'$$

which implies $\mathsf{MX}_0 = 0$, then maximize

$$l' = -\log(\det(\mathsf{MVM})) - (\mathsf{MY})'(\mathsf{MVM})^{-1}\mathsf{MY}.$$

The variance components can be estimated from maximizing l' and $\hat{\mathsf{b}}_0$ given by (1) provides an estimator of β_0. Finally, N_i in (2) yields an asymptotically normally distributed test statistic for the hypothesis of no group effect.

There is no categorical answer as to whether the ordinary or the restricted maximum likelihood estimators should be preferred. However, the restricted maximum likelihood method has the advantage of yielding unbiased estimators of the variance components in the case of balanced designs.

4 Discussion and a Numerical Example

To provide a numerical example for the methods described so far we analyzed an embryotoxicity study which consisted of two groups with 15 rabbits in each group. In table 1 the unweighted means of the crown-rump length, the fetal weight and the placental weight are given. Table 2 summarizes the results for the fixed effects (FE), maximum likelihood (ML) and restricted maximum likelihood (REML) approach.

With the (generally invalid) FE-method, we get a significant difference for the fetal weights. ML and REML yield qualitatively the same results though REML is a little more conservative than ML. We do not know whether this can be said in a general context.

Parameter	Group 1 (87 obs.)	Group 2 (83 obs.)
Crown-rump length (mm)	96.34 ± 4.9	97.79 ± 3.7
Fetal weight (g)	40.51 ± 4.7	42.87 ± 3.9
Placental weight (g)	5.92 ± 0.9	5.62 ± 1.1

Table 1: Unweighted means and standard deviations.

Parameter	FE	ML	REML
Crown-rump length	0.235	0.341	0.360
Fetal weight	0.038*	0.089	0.103
Placental weight	0.551	0.543	0.568

Table 2: P-values for several kinds of analysis.

We can summarize the discussion of the present paper as follows:

- For the analysis of continuously distributed offspring data, tests based on least squares with known (finite) distributions do not exist.
- Tests based on likelihood methods are valid only asymptotically.
- Every procedure discussed so far relies on assumptions concerning the underlying distributions which may not hold in general.
- Nonparametric and/or robust alternatives do not seem to exist at present.

References

Gates, C.E., Chiue, C. (1962). The analysis of variance of the s-stage hierarchical model. *Biometrics* **18**, 529–536.

Gower, J.C. (1962). Variance component estimation for unbalanced hierarchical classifications. *Biometrics* **18**, 537–542.

Healy, M.J.R. (1972). Animal litters as experimental units. *Applied Statistics* **21**, 155–159.

SAS Institute Inc. (1988). *SAS/STAT User's Guide, Release 6.03 Edition.* Cary, NC: SAS Institute Inc.

Satterthwaite, F.E. (1946). An approximate distribution of estimates of variance components. *Biometrics Bulletin* **2**, 110–114.

Searle, S.R. (1987). *Linear Models for Unbalanced Data.* New York: John Wiley & Sons.

GENERAL STATISTICAL PRINCIPLES IN TESTING OF TOXICOLOGICAL STUDIES

Ludwig Hothorn
German Cancer Research Center, D-6900 Heidelberg

1. Introduction

To present an overview paper on the general principles of biostatistics in toxicology threatens to discuss insignificances, because statistics for toxicology in general do not exist. The field of toxicology includes a broad spectrum of different methods and problems.
This paper is limited to studies of the so-called regulatory toxicology: assays for the characterization of new chemicals, e.g., drugs, according to national or international guidelines (e.g., EC guideline for testing of drugs, anonymous, 1983) and regulations (e.g., GLP regulations of the OECD, anomymous, 1983a). For a clear discussion of some biostatistical methods, only one assay will be chosen here: a four week subchronic toxicity study on rats according to EC guidelines: $\{TREATMENT > TIME \ * \ SEX\}$
with treatment: Control, $Dose_1$, $Dose_2$, $Dose_3$
time: t_0, t_{28d}, t_{rev} sex: female, male
and several endpoints, e.g., body mass, hemoglobin etc. .

Furthermore this paper is directed at the problem of multiple comparisons in "Control versus k treatment or dose groups design":

* it represents the main problem in nearly all studies
* important developments on this topic in the last decade

2. The formulation of hypotheses

Studies of regulatory toxicology represent so-called "safety studies" ; the purpose of these studies is the **certain** registration of toxic, carcinogenic, teratogenic, and mutagenic **side-effects** of the substance under investigation (while the pharmacological main effect was

most likely investigated beforehand).
Based on this purpose, the formulation of the statistical testing hypotheses in relation to type I and II errors should be specified.

In classical statistics for the comparison between a control and a treatment group (in a two sample, one-sided case), the hypothesis can be formulated as:

null hypothesis: $F_C = F_T$
alternative hypothesis: $F_C < F_T$
with F_T ... distribution function of the treatment group

Decision scheme:

	H_0 *holds*	H_A *holds*
H_0 *will be accepted*	*correct*	*type II error* β
H_0 *will be rejected*	*type I error*	*correct*

The risk of a type I error represents the *producer's risk*: the conclusion that a toxic side-effect exists, while in truth this is not the case. The risk of a type II error represents the *customers's risk* the conclusion that no toxic side-effect exists, while in truth there does exist such a toxic effect. It is intuitively clear that it is necessary to handle both risks with care **but controlling the type II error rate should be of primary concern in toxicology** .

Between both risks, the following general relation holds (in the two-sample case):

$$\beta = f(\alpha, \sigma, 1/d, 1/n_j)$$

with σ ... variable specific variance
d ... detectable difference between control and treatment

But in the hypothesis formulation given above, the type I error can only be controlled directly (by choosing the related quantile of the test statistics). For the two-sample case this hypothesis formulation can be reversed to control α for a type II error, but for the usual k-sample design used in toxicological studies this results in complicated testing distributions.

Usually the type II error is defined comparisonwise, while the type I error is defined experimentwise .
Within a typical design, comparisons between:

- control and the treatment groups
- several time points
- both sexes
- and for a multivariate variable vector

should be analyzed. Because of the dramatic increase in the type II error with such a high-dimensional experimentwise α formulation, usually only for the sub-design "control versus k treatment or dose groups" the experimentwise alpha should be used.

Based on this formulation, the purpose of an adequate statistical analysis should be directed at:

Minimizing the type II error rate and holding the experimentwise type I error rate α_e (based on the sub-design "control versus treatments or dose groups)

The following chapters will address several methods of meeting this objective.

If this compromise is not possible in an approximate way, then methods with comparisonwise α should be used in toxicology to ensure an optimal power rather methods enforcing an experimentwise error rate but with the consequence of low power.

3. Experimental design

For the above mentioned sub-design three important types can be distinguished:

type 1) $\{Control, Dose_1, \ldots, Dose_k\}$

with $Control=Dose_0<Dose_1<\ldots<Dose_k$

The purpose is the analysis of the dose-response relationship or the estimation of the no-observed effect level (NOEL)

type 2) $\{Control, Treatment_1, \ldots, Treatment_k\}$

with treatment ... several substances, combinations,etc.

The purpose is the comparison between these treatments and the control only.

type 3) $\{Control, Treatment\ or\ dose\ groups, Positive\ Control\}$

The purpose of using a positive control consist in the actually proof of the sensitivity of the animal strain. To hold α_e for this special design, a special testing method according to Hothorn (1991) can be used.

4. Modelling versus testing

Depending on the design and the purpose of the toxicological study, two main types of statistical analysis can be performed:

Design	Purpose	Method
type 1	dose-response analysis	modelling
	estimation of selected values based on a model	modelling
	low-dose extrapolation	modelling
	NOEL estimation	testing
	effect detection	testing
type 2	comparison of substances	testing
	effect estimation	testing

Examples of modelling in toxicology:

* model for the Ames-assay according to Margolin et al. (1981)
* multistage model in carcinogenesis according to Armitage (1982)

For the subchronic study mentioned above, both methods are possible; in the case of NOEL estimation based on a model the type II error may be smaller than with testing, provided the model is adequate. But in the possible case of an inadequate model the error may be greater. The biostatistical literature demonstrates how complicated it is to find an adequate model for the simple case of the AMES assay (see e.g., Edler and Vollmar, 1991). For routine evaluation of chronic toxicity studies with several variables such a model choice is rather difficult in practice. Because of this dependence of the type II error on the correctness of the a priori assumption of the model structure, **only testing will be discussed here.**

5. Testing in the "control versus k treatment or dose groups design"

5.1. Two-sample versus k-sample testing

In the toxicological literature the two-sample t-or Wilcoxon-Mann-Whitney(WMW)-U-test is also commonly used in "control versus k treatment or dose groups design", e.g., Jossan et al. (1989). Because of the violation of the experimentwise alpha formulation, this method should be avoided, even if in this case the type II error can be smaller than in the k-sample analysis. Comparison procedures "control versus k treatments or dose groups design", which controls α_e should be used.

If two-sample tests are nevertheless used, then only the comparisons between the control and the dose groups should be analyzed but not between the dose groups.

Example: Estimations of α_j for $k=3$, $n_j=16$ and $\alpha_e=0.05$

two-sample tests	*two-sample tests*	*k-sample procedure*
$C-D_j$	$C-D_j$ & D_j-D_i	*"control versus k doses"*
$\alpha/3$	$\alpha/6$	
0.0167	*0.0083*	*0.0199*

5.2. k-sample tests versus k-sample procedures

A k-sample test represents a single decision problem:

$$H_0: \; F_C = F_{T1} = \ldots\ldots = F_{Tk}$$

$$H_A: \; F_C \neq F_{T1} \neq \ldots\ldots \neq F_{Tk}$$

for testing the global substance effect in the k-sample design, while a comparison procedure represents a multiple decision problem: $H_A: \; F_i \neq F_j \quad i,j \in (1,\ldots,k)$

for testing every comparison.

In toxicological studies interest typically lies not only the global effect, but also in each comparison control versus $dose_j$, so that commonly k-sample procedures "control versus k treatment or dose group design", like Dunnett's (1955) procedure should be used.

With the closed testing methodology both methods can be combined (Hothorn, 1990):

Example with the above study : Control with 3 dose groups

Test statistic : parametric trend test according to (Fligner and Wolfe, 1982) for "control versus k dose groups design"

Testing strategy:

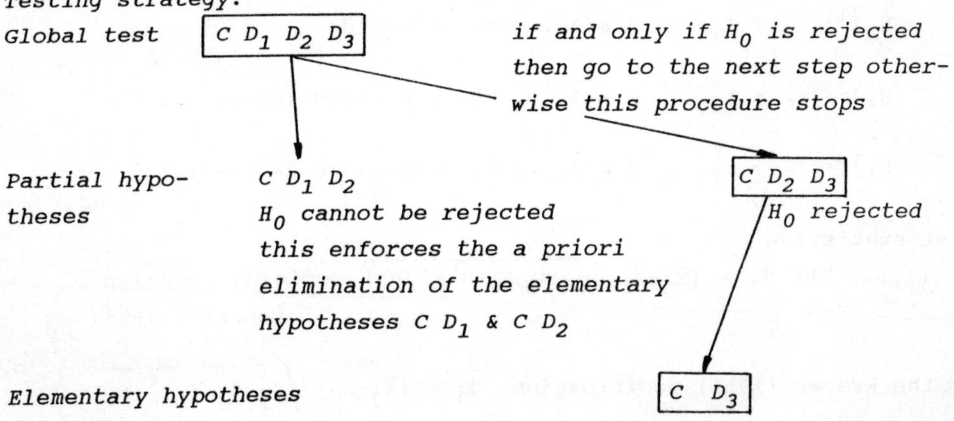

With this strategy both the k-sample test and the single comparisons C-D_j can be analyzed.

5.3. All-pair procedures versus "control versus k treatment or dose groups design" procedures

In the commonly used statistical software packages, all-pair comparison procedures like Tukey, Duncan and Scheffe procedures are available. Here not only the comparison between control and treatment groups will be performed but also between all treatment groups. In relation to procedures for "control versus k treatments or dose group design", there exists an increase in the type II error probability, increasing with higher dimensions of k.

Example: Control versus 3 dose groups (α_e*=0.05,* σ/d *=1.0,* n_j*=24)*

All-pair procedure	*"Control versus k dose groups"procedure*
Tukey procedure	*Dunnett procedure*
β*=0.200*	β*=0.106*

5.4. Dunnett's (1955) procedure

In "control versus k treatments or dose groups designs" Dunnett's procedure for approximately normally distributed variables is commonly used to control the level. Hypotheses:

$H_O \;: F_C = F_{Tj} \quad j \in (1,...,k)$

$H_A{}^{j1}: F_C \neq F_{Tj} \quad j \in (1,...,k)$ two-sided

$H_A{}^{j2}: F_C < F_{Tj} \quad j \in (1,...,k)$ one-sided increasing

$H_A{}^{j3}: F_C > F_{Tj} \quad j \in (1,...,k)$ one-sided decreasing

Test statistics

j (1,...,k): $d_j = (\bar{x}_j - \bar{x}_C)/\sqrt{MQ_R(1/n_C + 1/n_j)}$ original version (Dunnett, 1955)

or the Kramer (1956) modification $d_j = (\bar{x}_j - \bar{x}_C)/\sqrt{s_j^2/n_j + s_C^2/n_C}$

$$\text{with } MQ_R = \left(\sum_{j=C}^{k} \sum_{i=1}^{nj} x_{ij} - \left(\sum_{j=C}^{k} x_{j.}^2/n_j\right)\right) / \sum_{j=C}^{k}(n_j-1) \text{ mit } j \in (C,1,\ldots,k)$$

Decision rule:

The alternative hypothesis H_A^{j1} will be accepted, if

$d_j > d_{k,df,cj,1-}$,two-sided with $df = \sum_{j=C}^{k}(n_j-1)$ with $j \in (C,1,\ldots,k)$

with $c_j = 1/\sqrt{(n_j/n_C+1)}$

The alternative hypothesis H_A^{j2} will be accepted , if

$d_j > d_{k,df,cj,1-\alpha}$,one-sided

The alternative hypothesis H_A^{j3} will be accepted, if

$-d_j > d_{k,df,cj,1-\alpha}$,one-sided

The quantiles of the multivariate t-distribution (for equal correlation coefficients c_j) $d_{k,df,1-\alpha,direction}$ are tabled in Dunnett (1955); Dunnett (1964) and Ahner and Passing (1983). The quantiles of the multivariate t distribution for any correlation coefficients c_j are tabled in Gupta et al. (1985) or computer programs are available: Ahner and Passing (1983) and Hothorn and Spantig (1986).

Note 1: According to Rudolph (1988) Dunnett's procedure is relatively robust against violation of the normal distribution assumption; however for n_j >10 the non-parametric Steel (1959) procedure shows smaller type II errors .

Note 2: According to Horn (1979) minimum type II errors are attaint with sample sizes $n_K = \sqrt{k}\, n_j$.

Note 3: The type II errors depend on k, which implies that inclusions of further non-significant treatment groups can significant effects to be overlooked.

Example: Serum-ASAT-values in mol/ls, one-sided test of increase

Control	*Dose 1 20 mg/kg*	*Dose 2 200 mg/kg*	*Dose 3 1000 mg/kg*	
2.087	*2.064*	*2.515*	*2.649*	$\bar{x}_j$
.569	*.304*	*.722*	*.831*	s_j
	-.106	*2.048*	*2.499*	d_j
	2.14	*2.14*	*2.14*	$d_{k=3,df=36,1-\alpha=.95}$
	-	-	>	*result*

Inclusion of a non-significant low dose group

	low-dose	Dose1	Dose 2	Dose 3	
Control	10 mg/kg	20 mg/kg	200 mg/kg	1000 mg/kg	
2.087	2.072	2.064	2.515	2.649	$\bar{x}_j$
.569	.491	.304	.722	.831	s_j
	-.071	-.106	2.048	2.499	d_j
	2.55	2.55	2.55	2.55	$d_{k=4,1-\alpha=.95}$
	-	-	-	-	result

Due to the effect of including a non-significant low-dose group, the minimal number of treatments or dose groups necessary should be chosen during the experimental design of a new study. However, studies with as many as 16 groups have been described in the literature (Peto et al., 1984).

Note 4: In the case of variance heterogeneity, Dunnett's procedure is not robust according to Rudolph (1988) and Hothorn (1987). For small dimensions of k , e.g. the typical values k=3 or 4, the application of the Holm-Bonferroni adjusted (see chapter 5.5) Welch-t two sample test may be a good alternative, because even in the case of homogenous variances the type II error rates of this modification are not more important :

e.g. case $k=3, \alpha=0.05, n_j=10, s=16$ *ASAT values*

Expected values				Dunnett procedure			adjust. Welch-t		
μ_C	μ_1	μ_2	μ_3	β_1	β_2	β_3	β_1	β_2	β_3
60	80	90	100	.37	.06	.02	.19	.04	.02
60	75	85	95	.63	.17	.02	.41	.13	.02
60	80	100	100	.30	.01	.01	.19	.01	.01
60	75	75	100	.63	.63	.01	.41	.45	.99

5.5. Simultaneous versus sequential rejection procedures

One of the important modification of multiple decision problems consists in the closed testing methodology according to Marcus et al., (1976). The modification of multiple comparison procedures in "control versus k treatments or dose groups design " is particularly simple, because according to Sonnemann (1982) these represent a complete system of hypotheses of $(2^k -1)$ elementary hypotheses.

Control versus k treatments or dose groups procedures can be modified in four ways:

a) Bonferroni-Holm (1979) α-adjustment based on two-sample tests, e.g. the Welch test described above

b) sequential rejection modification according to Marcus et al., (1976)

c) Hommel (1988)/Hochberg(1988) "reverse Holm procedure" based on two-sample tests

d) closed testing procedure based on global tests, e.g., Fligner/ Wolfe (1982) trend test or Dunnett-max-test according to Hothorn (1990)

a) Bonferroni-Holm-procedure

For the elementary hypotheses $\{C-D_j\}$, specific two-sample tests are used (e.g. t-test or WMW-Test) and the following decision scheme according to the ordered p-values $p_{(j)}$: $p_{(1)} < p_{(2)} < \ldots < p_{(k)}$

if $p_{(1)} > \alpha/k$ ---> STOP, $H_0^{(1)}, \ldots, H_0^{(k)}$ are valid

↓ no

if $p_{(2)} > \alpha/(k-1)$ ---> STOP, $H_A^{(1)}, H_0^{(2)}, \ldots, H_0^{(k)}$ are valid

↓ no etc.

b) Marcus-modification

Step 1: Computation of all $j \in (1,\ldots,k)$ test statistics

$$d_j = (\bar{x}_j - \bar{x}_C) / \sqrt{MQ_R(1/n_C + 1/n_j)}$$

Step 2: Ordering to: $d_{(1)} \le d_{(2)} \le \ldots \le d_{(k)}$

Step 3: decision scheme

if $d_{(k)} < d_{k,FG,1-\alpha}$ ---> stop, H_0^{global} is valid

↓ no

if $d_{(k-1)} < d_{k-1,FG,1-\alpha}$ ---> stop, $H_A^{((k))}$ and $H_0^{((k-1),\ldots,(1))}$ are valid etc.

↓ no

c) Hommel-Hochberg-procedure

For the elementary hypotheses $\{K-D_j\}$, specific two-sample tests are used (e.g. t-test or WMW-Test) and the following decision scheme according to the ordered p-values $p_{(j)}$: $p_{(1)} < p_{(2)} < \ldots < p_{(k)}$

if $p_{(k)} < \alpha$ ---> all $H_0^{(1)}, \ldots, H_0^{(k)}$ are rejected & stop otherwise $H_0^{(k)}$ is valid , go to the next step

↓

if $p_{(k-1)} < \alpha/2$ ---> etc.

↓

if $p_{(j)} < \alpha/(k-j+1)$ otherwise go to the next step

d) closed testing procedure (see chapter 5.2.)

Example (data see above)

a) Bonferroni/Holm-procedure

$p_1 = -.106 \quad p_2 = .024 \quad p_3 = .001$
$p_{(1)} = .001 < p_{(2)} = .024 < p_{(3)} = .600$
$p_{(1)} < \alpha/k = 0.05/3 = 0.0166 \quad H_A^{(1)}$ is valid --->
$p_{(2)} = .024 < \alpha/(k-1) = .025 \quad H_A^{(2)}$ is valid --->
$p_{(3)} = .600 > \alpha/(k-2) = .05 \quad H_0^{(3)}$ is valid & stop.

* Original Bonferroni-procedure

$t_1 = -.106 \quad t_2 = 2.048 \quad t_3 = 2.499$
$p_1 = .60 \quad p_2 = .024 \quad p_3 = .001$
$p_{(1)} = .001 < p_{(2)} = .024 < p_{(3)} = .600$
with $p_{(1)} = .001 < \alpha/k = .05/3 = .0167 \quad H_A^{(1)}$ is valid --->
with $p_{(2)} = .024 > \alpha/k = .05/3 = .0167 \quad H_0^{(2)}$ is valid and stop.

b) Marcus-modification

$d_{(1)} = -.106 < d_{(2)} = 2.048 < d_{(3)} = 2.499$
$d_{3,FG=36,1-\alpha=.95} = 2.14 < d_{(3)}$ $(K\text{-}D_3)$ there is a significant difference --->
$d_{2,FG=36,1-\alpha=.95} = 1.98 < d_{(2)}$ $(K\text{-}D_2)$ there is a significant difference --->
$d_{1,FG=36,1-\alpha=.95} = 1.69 > d_{(1)}$ $(K\text{-}D_1)$ no difference & stop

c) Hommel-Hochberg-procedure

$p_{(3)} = .60 > .05 \quad H_0^{(3)}$ is valid, go to the next step
$p_{(2)} = .024 < 0.05/2 \quad H_A^{(2)}$ and $H_A^{(1)}$ are valid.

d) Closed testing procedure based on Dunnett-max-test

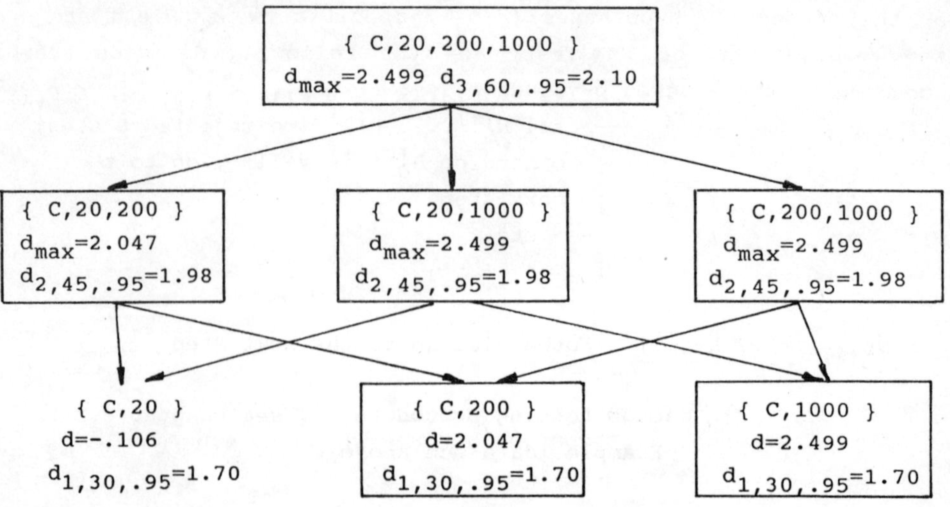

In the sense of the above conclusions on minimizing type II errors, these modified procedures should be recommended in general, but for these conditional single comparisons the computation of *simultaneous confidence intervals* is not possible.

Significance testing gives information only on the acceptance or rejection of any null hypothesis , but not about the extent of the deviation from of the null hypothesis. This is possible with simultaneous confidence intervals concerning the differences of the expected values $\mu_j - \mu_C$ e.g. of Dunnett's procedure:

$$[\ \bar{x}_j-\bar{x}_C-d_{k,df,1-\alpha}\sqrt{MQR(1/n_j+1/n_C)}\ ;\ \bar{x}_j-\bar{x}_C+d_{k,df,1-\alpha}\sqrt{MQR(1/n_j+1/n_C)}\ ]$$

5.6. Non-restricted alternative hypotheses versus ordered alternative hypotheses

Now we consider experimental design type 1 only: C, $Dose_1, \ldots, Dose_k$ With the restriction on the alternative hypothesis of a monotonic ordering, a reduction of the type II error probability may be possible

$$H_A : \quad F_C \le F_{D1} \le \ldots \le F_{Dk} \quad \text{with at least} \quad F_C < F_{Dk}$$

For "control versus k dose groups design" the Williams (1971) procedure is the analogous to the Dunnett-procedure with an ordered alternative. For monotonic dose-response relationships in a simulation study, the advantages with respect to type II error rates can be shown clearly (Hothorn, 1989):

Example: $k = 3\ \alpha = 0.05\ n_j = 5\ \sigma^2 = 1$

Typ	*expected value profile*				*Dunnett-procedure*			*Williams-procedure*		
	μ_C	μ_{D1}	μ_{D2}	μ_{D3}	β_1	β_2	β_3	β_1	β_2	β_3
mono-	*0*	*0*	*.2*	*1*	*.997*	*.916*	*.241*	*.970*	*.853*	*.144*
ton	*0*	*.33*	*.66*	*1*	*.835*	*.513*	*.149*	*.737*	*.365*	*.056*
	0	*.5*	*1*	*1*	*.731*	*.238*	*.246*	*.626*	*.164*	*.074*
non-	*0*	*.5*	*1*	*.5*	*.650*	*.124*	*.650*	*.542*	*.194*	*.190*
monoton	*0*	*1*	*.5*	*1*	*.249*	*.740*	*.246*	*.351*	*.335*	*.104*

In this table the advantage of type II errors of the procedure an with ordered alternative in relation to the procedure with an unrestricted alternative, even in the case of small non-monotonicities. In the case of marked non-monotonocity, so-called umbrella alternatives, these procedures with ordered alternatives are non-robust (Hothorn, 1987) and tests/procedures with non-restricted alternatives or special tests/procedures for these umbrella alternatives should be used (e.g., for the analysis of the Ames-assay: (Gretzebach et al., 1988; Rothe, 1985).

Another simple procedure with an ordered alternative is based on the principle of a priori ordering of hypotheses of interest according to Maurer (1987). In a k-sample problem the $(H^1,\ldots,H^k)$ pairs of hypotheses $\{H_0 ; H_A\}$ can be divided in two groups G1 = $(H^1,\ldots,H^i)$ and G2 = $(H^{i+1},\ldots,H^k)$ in such a way that the hypotheses in group G2 are only interesting, if and only if, all null hypotheses in group G1 were rejected.

The hypotheses in group G1 are to be tested with methods which control the multiple α level without considering group G2. If and only if, all null hypotheses in group G1 were rejected, then the hypotheses in group G2 can be tested with a multiple method on the same significance level. All implications of the null-hypotheses of the group G1 which are also implications of null-hypotheses in group G2 can be considered as a priori rejected. This principle controls the multiple α level for the whole procedure (for proof see Maurer, 1987).

Here a modification for more than two groups G^j and one-sided ordered alternatives in "control versus k treatments" design is given :

* In a k-sample problem with one-sided ordered alternatives we form k ordered groups of hypotheses pairs $G^{(j)}$, so that $G^{(j-1)}$ (with $j \in (k,\ldots,1)$) is of interest if and only if, the null-hypothesis $H_0^{(j)}$ was rejected.
* Because "control versus k treatments designs" represent a complete family of hypotheses, no implications of hypotheses between the groups $G^{(j)}$ exist.
* Procedure: $G^{(k)}$: testing $H_0^{(k)}$ with a two sample test "control versus treatments k" on level α. If $H_0^{(k)}$ is valid, all $H_0^{(k,\ldots,1)}$ hold and the procedure stops If $H_0^{(k)}$ is rejected, $H_A^{(k)}$ holds; continuation with $G^{(k-1)}$

  $G^{(k-1)}$: testing $H_0^{(k-1)}$ with a two sample test "control versus treatment k-1" on level α; and so on, possible down to $G^{(1)}$

Another view of this procedure is given by a subset of the closed testing procedure for "control versus k treatment" designs for one-sided ordered alternative, where the j-sample trend test with j (k,...,1) was substituted by a one-sided two sample test $\{C\text{-}D_j\}$.

The choice of the two sample tests is flexible and depends on the kind of variable (see chapter 5.8.).
The behaviour of the procedure (designated as EAP), based on a multiple t-test as an example, was characterized in relation to the Williams and the Dunnett procedures by simulation for several distributions, expected values profiles, sample sizes and levels (Hothorn, 1990a); here are only presented some estimations of type II errors:

Expected value profile	Williams			EAP			Dunnett		
μ_C μ_1 μ_2 μ_3	$\hat{\beta}_3$	$\hat{\beta}_2$	$\hat{\beta}_1$	$\hat{\beta}_3$	$\hat{\beta}_2$	$\hat{\beta}_1$	$\hat{\beta}_3$	$\hat{\beta}_2$	$\hat{\beta}_1$
0 0 .2 1	.135	.853	.970	.134	.861	.978	.241	.916	.977
0 .33 .66 1	.056	.365	.764	.071	.396	.782	.149	.513	.835
0 .5 1 1	.074	.164	.626	.174	.233	.645	.246	.238	.731
0 .5 .5 1	.047	.465	.600	.064	.556	.695	.107	.686	.650

With simulations it was shown that this procedure is relatively robust for moderate non-monotonic dose-response relationships (Hothorn, 1990a). The EAP-procedure is recommended in the case of "in general monotone dose-response relationships" because the use of any simple two-sample tests is possible.

5.7. Normal distribution assumption versus mixing distribution assumption

All methods discussed above are directed at testing expected values (or approximate mean values) only, with the assumption of equal variances. In real toxicological studies a greater variability with increasing mean response is not unusual. There are several methods to treat this problem:

* adjustment of the test statistics in the direction of the homoge neity case , e.g., see above WELCH-t test
* simultaneous testing of location and scale alternatives with so-called location-scale models, e.g., in the non-parametric case a statistic, consisting of a linear combination of WMW test for location and Ansari/Bradley (1960) test for scale according to Lepage (1971).
* Sometimes this variability may be due to the presence of "non-responders" in the treatment groups. Analogous to the acute toxicity model, (1-p) animals can control their behaviour under substance action (they survived, like untreated animals ="non-responder", p other animals however cannot be controlled, they react pathologically or die (= responder).

Such examples were given in the literature by Garby et al.(1969) for a nutrition study, by Nation et al. (1984) for a behavioural toxicological study, by Cory-Slechta et al. (1981) for a teratological study, by Johnson et al. (1987) for sister chromatid exchange (mutagenicity assay), by Good (1979) for a pharmacological study and by Conover and Salsburg (1988) for a clinical trial. The common analysis in toxicology with mean values can lead to misinterpretation in the sense of "the cow drowned in the in average 70 cm deep lake".

The following statistical model will be considered here:

Let $X_1, \ldots, X_m$ be the responses of the control with the distribution function H(x), and $Y_1, \ldots, Y_n$ the responses of a treatment group with the distribution function G(x). The hypothesis can be formulated as:

$H_O \; : \; H(x) = G(x)$

$H_A \; : \; H(x) \neq G(x) \qquad$ with $G(x) = (1-p)H(x)+pF_{patho}$

with p...unknown (1-p) non-responder p responder

shift : $H_A^1 \quad F_{patho} = H(x-d)$ here one-sided alternative with $d > 0$ (Good, 1979)

power type 1 $H_A^2 \quad F_{patho} = H^a(x)$ (Lehmann, 1953)

power type 2 $H_A^3 \quad F_{patho} = (1-(1-H^{1/a}))$ (Conover and Salsburg, 1988)

(Good, 1979) proposed a randomization test for H_A^1, for which (Boos and Brownie, 1980) published a modification. (Johnson et al.,1987) suggested approximative score statistics based on a mixed normal score function:

$$sm(4) = \exp(-d^2/2)\exp(d\varnothing^{-1}(u))-1 \qquad 0 < u < 1$$

and a quantile test based on bi-uniform score function. (Conover and Salsburg, 1988) proposed a modified t-test based on approximate score functions:

$$scs(i) = (i/(N+1))^{a-1}$$

with i ... rank in the combined (x+y) sample for hypothesis H_A^2 and

$$sc(i) = -\ln(1-i/(n+1)) \quad \text{for the hypothesis } H_A^3.$$

In a simulation study, the behaviour of some tests under Lehmann alternatives was investigated (Hothorn, 1991a). Here only for selected conditions the comparison of the ß estimations of t-test and an optimal scores test will be given in figure 1.

At present these score procedures should be used in toxicology in an explorative way only.

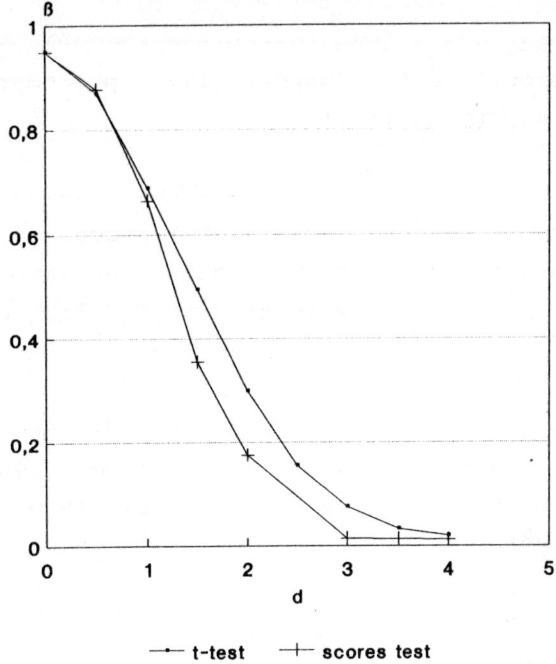

5.8. Types of variables and types of procedures

Not only continuous, approximately normally distributed variables like body mass or hemoglobin concentration will be measured in toxicological studies, but also many other types. It is desirable to perform the analysis of all these types of variables with the same methodology for "control versus k treatment or dose groups design". In the following table for selected variables related comparison procedures for the one-way design "control versus k treatment or dose groups" for restricted or unrestricted alternative hypotheses are given.

ordered alternative	**non-restricted alternative**
Williams (1971)-procedure[1)] or EAP-procedure according to Hothorn (1991)	Dunnett (1955)-procedure[1)2)]
Shirley (1977)-procedure[1)] modification according to Williams (1986) or EAP-procedure[2)] based on WMW-test	Steel (1959)-procedure[1)] or Dunnett (1955)-procedure with data transformation according to Conover and Salsburg (1988)
Shirley (1977)-procedure[1)] with correction for ties or EAP-procedure[2)], based on WMW test with ties correction according to Büning and Trenkler (1978)	Ahner and Passing (1983) modification of Steel (1959) procedure[1)2]
Closed testing version of Armitage (1955) test or EAP-Procedure,based on approx. Fisher-test acc. to Gart et al. (1986)	Passing (1984)-procedure[1)]
Closed testing version of Lee (1985) trend test or EAP procedure based on test acc. to Kalbfleish [1)] and Sprott (1973) acc. to Hothorn (1990)	procedure "control versus k treatments" for Poisson-distributed variables accord. Hothorn (1989b)

1) As sequential rejection modification according to Hothorn (1989b)

2) As a Lehmann-alternative-test version with data transformation

type of variable	**example**	**class of statistics**
contin., approx. normally dist.	Hemoglobin	parametric statistics
contin., non-normally dist.	Alkaline Phosphatase	for n<10 parametric procedure for n>10 non-parametric procedure
discrete, large numbers	Erythrocytes	non-parametric procedure with correction for ties
proportion (dichotomous)	number tied/number all animals	comparison procedure for proportions
number of findings (countable)	number of tumours	comparison procedure for Poisson-distributed variables

5.10. Selection criteria for comparison procedures in "control versus k treatment or dose group designs" in toxicological studies

In the above chapters many details for the application of optimal comparison procedures for "control versus k treatment or dose group designs" were discussed in the sense of minimizing type II error rates while controlling experimentwise alpha level.
Some recommendations will be briefly given:

* *decide between modelling and testing; for routine analysis only testing will be recommended (and discussed)here*
* *use comparison procedures instead of two-sample tests*
* *use comparison procedure "control versus k treatment or dose groups" instead of all-pair procedures*
* *use comparison procedures instead of k-sample tests; even more preferable is the combination of both in sense of closed testing procedure*
* *use specific comparison procedures related to the type of variable*
* *for n>10 use the non-parametric STEEL procedure, even under the normal distribution assumption*
* *use the optimal sample size design:* $n_C = \sqrt{k} n_j$
* *use the lowest possible number of treatment/dose groups k within a simultaneous analysis*
* *use a sequential rejection modification or a closed testin procedure instead of a simultaneous procedure, but not if confidence intervals are of interest*
* *for the design* $Control<Dose_1<...<Dose_k$, *use procedures with ordered alternative hypotheses e.g. Williams/Shirley procedure (or EAP); these are robust against moderate violations of the monotonicity assumption*
* *in the case of simultaneous effects of mean values and variances, use comparison procedures based on scores for so-called Lehmann alternatives or for adjustment of the heterogeneity effect only the Holm-Bonferroni-Welch-t test*
* *use a multivariate analysis based on a closed testing procedure of multiple endpoint analysis for p<6 preselected variables* [1)]

For practical application these recommendations are unfortunally somewhat "theoretical", because in the commonly used software packages these methods are not available; only the PC-program HI-TOX (Hothorn, Spantig and Nagel, 1989) contains these modules.

1) A chapter on multivariate testing in toxicology was eliminated in this book, see Hothorn (1991a).

6. Summary

In this overview paper, an attempt was made to formulate the general purpose of biostatistical methods in toxicology. These methods were demonstrated using a simple subchronic toxicity study. The emphasis was the testing with comparison procedures in the one-way design "control versus k treatment or dose groups".
Many other aspects were not discussed here, e.g. the analysis of mortality or tumour-time responses (see e.g., GART et al., 1986), analysis of the effects of combined substances (see e.g., Unkelbach and Wolf, 1988), analysis of time-series or multifactor designs, etc. This paper and this workshop in general should stimulate thinking about the sophisticated biostatistical problems in toxicology and further research in this area.

7. References

Ahner C and Passing H.(1983) Berechnung der multivariaten t-Verteilung und simultane Vergleiche gegen Kontrolle bei ungleichen Gruppenbesetzungen. EDV Med. Biolog. 14, 113-120.

anonymous (1983) Empfehlungen des Rates vom 26.10.83 zu den Versuchen mit Arzneispez. im Hinblick auf deren Inverkehrbringung. (83/571/ EWG).In: Pharmazeut. Industrie 45, 1248 - 1261.

anonymous (1983a) Bekanntmachung der OECD-Grundsätze der guten Laborpraxis (GLP). In: Pharma.Ind. 45, 260-265.

Ansari AR and Bradley RA (1960) Rank-sum tests for dispersions. Ann. Math.Stat. 31, 1174-1189.

Armitage P (1955) Tests for linear trends in proportions and frequencies. Biometrics 11, 375-386.

Armitage P (1982) The assessment of low-dose carcinogenicity. Biometrics,Suppl.:Current Topics in Biostatistics and Epidemiology, 38,119-129.

Boos DD and Brownie C (1986) Testing for a treatment effect in the presence of nonresponders. Biometrics 42, 191-197.

Büning H and Trenkler G (1978) Nichtparametrische statistische Methoden. W. de Gruyter, Berlin.

Conover WJ and Salsburg DS (1988) Locally most powerful tests for detecting treatment effects when a subset of patients can be expected to "respond" to treatment. Biometrics 44, 189-196.

Cory-Slechta DA et al. (1981) Chronic postweaning lead exposure and response duration performance. Tox.Appl.Pharm. 60, 78-84.

Dunnett CW (1955) A multiple comparison procedure for comparing several treatments with a control. JASA 50, 1096-1121.

Dunnett CW (1964) New tables for multiple comparisons with a control.

Biometrics 20, 560 - 572.

Edler L and Vollmar J (1991) Biostatistical issues in short-term tests for genetic toxicology. (Submitted)

Fligner MA and Wolfe DA (1982) Distrubution-free tests for comparing several treatments with a control. Statist.Neerl. 36, 119-127.

Garby L et al. (1969) Iron deficieny in women of fertile age in a Swedish community. Acta Med. Scand. 185, 113-117.

Gart JJ et al.(1986) The design and analysis of long-term animal experiments. IARC Sci. Publ. No. 79. Lyon, France.

Good PI (1979) Detection of a treatment effect when not all experimental subjects will respond to treatment. Biometrics 35, 483-489.

Gretzebach,L., Hothorn,L., Liese,F.: A simulation study for comparing test under umbrella alternatives, Probl.angew.Statist. (1988) 24, 55-68.

Gupta SS et al. (1985) On the distribution of the studentized maximum of equally correlated normal variables. Commum.Stat.B14, 103-135.

Hochberg Y (1988) A sharper Bonferroni procedure for multiple tests of significance. Biometrika 75, 800-803.

Holm S (1979) A simple sequentially rejective multiple test procedure. Scand. J. Statist. 6, 65 - 70.

Hommel G (1988) A stagewise rejective multiple test procedure based on a modified Bonferroni test. Biometrika 75, 383-386.

Horn M (1979) Regarding the optimality of the formula .. . Biometr.J. 21, 407-412.

Hothorn L (1987) k-Stichprobentests und -vergleichsprozeduren in Dosis-Wirkungs-Abhängigkeiten toxikologischer Untersuchungen. Habilschrift Universität Halle.

Hothorn L (1989) Robustness study on Williams and Shirley procedure, with applicat. in toxicology. Biometr.J. 31,891-903.

Hothorn L (1989a) On the behaviour of Fligner/Wolfe trend test "Control versus k treatments", with application in toxicology, Biometr Journ. 31, 767-780.

Hothorn L (1989b) A simple statistical procedure for testing tumour rates in animal carcinogenicity experiments. Arch. Toxicol.,Suppl. 13, 265-268.

Hothorn L (1990) Biometrische Analyse spezieller Untersuchungen der regulativen Toxikologie.In: Horn,M. und Hothorn,L.: Grundlagen der Statistik für Toxikologen. Verlag Volk.u.Gesundheit,Berlin.

Hothorn (1990a) A simple testing procedure "control versus k treatments" for one-sided ordered alternatives, with application in toxicology. Biometr. J. 33 (submitted).

Hothorn L (1991) Analysis of experimental designs with a positive control group in toxicology. Fundam.Appl.Tox. (submitted)

Hothorn L (1991a) Simulation study on tests with Lehmann alternatives (1991a) (in Vorbereitung)

Hothorn L and Spantig J.-U., (1986) Eine FORTRAN-Bibliothek wichtiger Pruefverteilungen auf Mikrorechner. Paper, 8. Biometr. Colloq. DDR-Region Inter.Biometr.Soc., Reinhardsbrunn.

Hothorn,L., Spantig,J.-U. and Nagel,M (1990) STATTOX, Version 2.0, Programmdokumentation.

Hothorn,L. and Nagel,M (1990) Hochinteraktive graphische Analyse multivariater Daten aus Toxikologie,Klinik und Epidem.(in Vorbereitung

Johnson RA et al. (1987) Two-sample rank tests for detecting changes that occur in small proportions of the treated population. Biometrics 43, 641-655.

Jossan SS et al. (1989) MPTP toxicity in relation to age, dopamine uptake and MAO-B activity in two rodent species. Pharmacol & Toxicol. 64, 314-318.

Kalbfleish JG Sprott DA (1973) The comparison of poisson-distributed oberservations. Biometrics 29, 223-224.

Kramer CY (1956) Extension of multiple range tests to group means with unequal numbers of replication. Biometrics 12, 307-310.

Lee YJ (1985) Tests in trends in Poisson means. J.Qual.Techn.17,44-49.

Lehmann EL (1953) Ther power of rank tests. Ann.Math.Statist. 24 (1953), 23-43.

Lepage Y (1971) A combination od Wilcoxon's and Ansari-Bradley's statistics. Biometrika 58, 231-217.

Marcus R et al.(1976) On closed testing procedures with special reference to ordered analysis of variance. Biometrika 63, 655 - 660.

Margolin BH et al. (1981) Statistical analysis of the Ames Salmonella/microsome test. Proc. Nat.Acad.Sci. 78,3779-3783.

Maurer W (1987) Statistische Besonderheiten bei klinischen Studien. Paper ROeS Intern.Biometr.Soc., Locarno.

Nation JR et al. The effects of oral cadmium exposure on a passive avoidance performance. Toxicol.Letters 20, 41-47.

Passing H (1984) Exact simultaneous comparisons with control in a r*c contingency table. Biometr. J. 26, 643-654.

Peto R et al. (1984) Nitrosoamine carcinogens in 5120 rodents. In: O'Neill IK ed.: N-Nitroso Compounds, IARC Sci.Publ. No.57,Lyon, 627-665.

Rothe G (1985) Zur statistischen Auswertung von Mutagenitätsexperimenten. Forschungsbericht 85/3 Universität Dortmund

Rudolph PE (1988) Robustness of multiple comparison procedures:Treatment versus control. Biometr.J. 30, 41-45.

Shirley EAC (1977) A non-parametric equivalent of Williams test for contrasting increasing dose levels of a treatment. Biometrics 33, 386-389.

Sonnemann E (1982) Allgemeine Lösungen multipler Testprobleme. EDV Med. Biolog. 13, 120-128.

Steel RGD (1959) A multiple comparison rank sum test treatment versus control, Biometrika 15: 560-572.

Unkelbach HD and Wolf Th (1983) Ehrlichkeit beim statistischen Testen. In: Vollmar J (ed.) Biometrie in der chemisch-pharmazeutischen Industrie, Vol.1,7-12. Fischer Verlag Stuttgart.

Williams DA (1971) A test for differences between treatment means when several dose levels are compared with a zero dose control. Biometrics 27, 103 - 117.

Williams DA (1986) A note on SHIRLEY's nonparametric test for comparing several dose levels with a zero-dose control. Biometrics 42, 183 - 186.

DETERMINATION OF ENDPOINTS IN ACUTE AND CHRONIC TOXICITY TESTS BY USING GENERALIZED LINEAR MODELS

Armand Maul

Département Informatique, Université de NANCY II,

boulevard Charlemagne 2, 54000 NANCY, France

Generalized linear models are suggested for regression analysis of dichotomous, count or continuous data. In particular, binomial, negative binomial and gamma regression analyses are shown to be interesting means for the determination of endpoints in toxicity tests. The process of model fitting, i.e., the maximum likelihood procedure, is developed by using a logistic function (binomial regression) or a log-linear regression model (negative binomial and gamma regression). Finally, inferences about various endpoints which are considered in acute and chronic toxicity tests are made and emphasized.

INTRODUCTION

Three kinds of data are usually obtained from bioassays, and more specifically, toxicity tests, namely: dichotomous (e.g., mortality), count (e.g., number of young) and continuous (e.g., weight) data.

For technical reasons arising from different application areas and objectives, different terminologies and computing tools have been developed for analyzing the three kinds of data (Gelber *et al.*, 1985). However, none of the conventional statistical procedures seems to be satisfactory for lack of generality, since most of the existing methods are characterized by the stringency of the underlying hypotheses and/or the subsequent narrowness of the areas in which they can be applied.

The purpose of this paper is to suggest some regression methods which can provide toxicologists with improved procedures for the determination of endpoints in toxicity tests. The probability distributions considered, namely: the binomial, the negative binomial or its limiting form (i.e., the Poisson) and the gamma distribution, are appropriate for dealing with a wide range of dichotomous, count and continuous data, respectively. Since all the previous distributions belong to the exponential family (Barndorff-Nielsen, 1978), the further developed techniques, herein called binomial, negative binomial and mixed Poisson, and gamma regression analysis, respectively, are special cases of the more general GLM theory (McCullagh and Nelder, 1983).

Further, the unknown parameters of the regression function, and subsequently the endpoint considered, can be estimated by using maximum likelihood methods. This is done under the assumption of a logistic function if binomial regression is performed whereas a log-linear regression model is used for modelling the association between the mean of the dependent variable and the explanatory variables in the regression analysis of count or continuous data.

STATISTICAL METHODS

. The models

Let $R_1, R_2, \ldots, R_n$ be a set of n random variables corresponding to independent observations. Three different assumptions are considered according as R_i $(i = 1,2,\ldots,n)$ follows:

1. a binomial distribution with parameters n_i and p_i

2 a) a negative binomial distribution with mean m_i and dispersion parameter k, or

b) its limiting form when k goes to infinity (i.e., the Poisson distribution with parameter m_i)

3. a gamma distribution with mean m_i and dispersion parameter k.

Note that k is assumed to be a constant (i.e., each of the n distributions considered in case 2 or 3 has the same dispersion parameter).

Given a set $x_1, x_2, \ldots, x_q$ of q explanatory variables, $(q < n)$ let us consider the models

$$p_i = 1 / (1 + \exp(\beta_1 x_{i1} + \beta_2 x_{i2} + \ldots + \beta_q x_{iq})) \qquad (1)$$

and

$$\ln m_i = \beta_1 x_{i1} + \beta_2 x_{i2} + \ldots + \beta_q x_{iq} \qquad (2)$$

where $x_{i1}, \ldots, x_{iq}$ are the values of $x_1, \ldots, x_q$ which are associated with the random variable R_i and $\beta_1, \ldots, \beta_q$ are the q unknown regression parameters.

Model (1), which expresses the probability p_i in the binomial distribution as a logistic function of the explanatory variables, is used when the response variable is binomial, whereas a linear function of the explanatory variables for modelling the natural logarithm of the mean m_i, as shown in model (2), is considered if R_i follows either a negative binomial or a gamma distribution. Regression analysis assuming these models will be referred to as binomial, negative binomial and mixed Poisson, and gamma regression, respectively. Note that within the present purpose, it is convenient and advisable to state $q = 3$ and $(x_{i1}, x_{i2}, x_{i3}) = (1, x_i, (x_i)^2)$ where x_i is the concentration level associated with the ith observation. Consequently, the linear part in models (1) and (2) is expressed as a quadratic function of the concentration x.

The use of binomial regression is suggested for analyzing dichotomous data which can, for example, be obtained in acute toxicity tests . On the other hand, both negative binomial and mixed Poisson regression, and also gamma regression are applicable to the statistical analysis of count and continuous data, respectively. These kinds of data may result from chronic toxicity experiments.

. Estimation of the parameters of the model

Let $\underline{\beta}$ be a column vector containing the unknown regression parameters β_1, β_2, β_3 of the model considered, and X the matrix of explanatory variables, with entries $x_{ij} = (x_i)^{j-1}$, i=1,....,n and j=1, 2, 3.

The maximum-likelihood estimates $\hat{\underline{\beta}}$ (resp. $(\hat{\underline{\beta}},\hat{k})$) of $\underline{\beta}$ (resp. $(\underline{\beta},k)$) for models (1) and (2) are obtained by maximizing the likelihood function $L(\underline{\beta})$ (resp. $L(\underline{\beta},k)$). Hence, the systems to be solved, under each of the previous assumptions are given as

$$X'.\,M_{(\underline{\beta})} = 0 \qquad \text{(binomial or Poisson)} \qquad \text{(3a)}$$

$$\begin{cases} X'.\,M_{(\underline{\beta})} = 0 \qquad \text{(negative binomial)} \qquad \text{(3b)} \\ D(k) = \sum_{i=1}^{n} \left[\left(\sum_{t=1}^{r_i} \frac{1}{k-1+t} \right) - \ln \left(1 + \frac{m_i}{k} \right) - \frac{r_i - m_i}{k + m_i} \right] = 0 \end{cases}$$

$$\begin{cases} X'.\, M_{(\underline{\beta})} = 0 \qquad \text{(gamma)} & \text{(3c)} \\ D(k) = n\left[\ln k - \dfrac{\Gamma'(k)}{\Gamma(k)}\right] + \displaystyle\sum_{i=1}^{n}\left[\left(1 - \dfrac{r_i}{m_i}\right) + \ln \dfrac{r_i}{m_i}\right] = 0 \end{cases}$$

where X' is the transpose of the matrix X, r_i the ith observation, and $M_{(\underline{\beta})}$ a column vector of length n with its ith term equal to

$n_i p_i - r_i$	(binomial)
$r_i - m_i$	(Poisson)
$(k(r_i - m_i))/(k + m_i)$	(negative binomial)
$k((r_i/m_i) - 1)$	(gamma)

according as binomial, Poisson, negative binomial or gamma regression analysis is performed, respectively.

Equations (3 a)b)c)) are nonlinear and their solution can be obtained by using an iterative procedure such as the Newton-Raphson method (Bard, 1974). This is quite easy for Equations (3a) or even the first three equations from System (3c) since the solution, as it appears immediately in the latter case, is independent from the value of the dispersion parameter k. As to the solution for Equations (3b), it is obtained by maximizing the likelihood function L, with respect to the β_j's (j = 1, 2, 3) for selected values of k (Lawless, 1987). This can be done by following a cross-iterative procedure which is based on the successive and alternate estimation of $\underline{\beta}$ and k (Maul *et al.*, 1990).

To this end, special computer programs have been written to carry out the estimation of all the parameters in Equations (3 a)b)c)). In addition to the estimation of $\underline{\beta}$, these programs provide maximum-likelihood estimates for the dispersion parameter in both the binomial and the gamma distribution.

The adequacy of models (1) and (2) for describing the data analyzed can be tested by means of a goodness-of-fit statistic which is -2 times the logarithm of the ratio of the likelihood for the current model to the likelihood of the saturated model (Nelder and Wedderburn, 1972).

. Estimation of endpoints

Assuming $f(x) = ß_1 + ß_2x + ß_3x^2$ is monotonic in such a way that $p = 1/(1 + \exp(f(x)))$ or $m = \exp(f(x))$ are decreasing functions of x on an interval $[a ; + \infty]$ $(a > 0)$, and regarding inferences about the various endpoints which are usually examined in toxicity tests, it is of interest to estimate the value x_r of the dose or the concentration level which corresponds to:

a) a prespecified value $p_r = 1/(1 + \exp(f(x_r)))$ $(0<p_r<1)$ of the probability p in model (1)

b) a prespecified relative variation , say a decrease by a rate 1 - r, given a specific value, x_s , of x, in the marginal mean m of the response variable in model (2) , regarding the corresponding mean m_s .

Denoting $\hat{ß}_1 + \hat{ß}_2x + \hat{ß}_3x^2$ by $\hat{f}(x)$ and $(1, x_r, (x_r)^2)$ by $\underline{x}_r$, it is easy to show that an estimate (and associated confidence limits at level $(1-\alpha)$) for x_r, in situation a), is given as

$$\hat{x}_r = \hat{f}^{-1} [\ln ((1/p_r) - 1)] \qquad (4)$$

(resp.) $$\hat{f}^{-1} [\ln ((1/p_r) - 1) \pm u_{(1-\alpha/2)}\sqrt{\mathrm{Var}\, [\underline{x}_r.\hat{\underline{ß}}]}\ ]$$

Situation a)

whereas, in situation b), an estimate (and corresponding confidence limits at level $(1-\alpha)$) for x_r is as follows

$$\hat{x}_r = \hat{f}^{-1} [\underline{x}_s.\hat{\underline{ß}} + \ln r]$$

(resp.) $$\hat{f}^{-1} [\underline{x}_s.\hat{\underline{ß}} + \ln r \pm u_{(1-\alpha/2)} \sqrt{\mathrm{Var}\, [\underline{x}_s.\hat{\underline{ß}}]}\ ]$$

Situation b)

where $\underline{x}_s.\hat{\underline{ß}}$ is the estimate of the marginal mean given x_s and $u_{(1-\alpha/2)}$ is obtained from the table of the standard normal distribution.

From a practical viewpoint, situation a) is applicable to acute toxicity tests for determining the effective dose level (e.g., the ED50) which corresponds to a prespecified quantile designated by p_r. The second situation refers more specifically to chronic toxicity tests. In particular, if $x_s = 0$, the value x_r is an estimate of the concentration of the test substance which is capable of inducing a relative inhibition by a rate 1-r from the control treatment on the biological attribute examined.

The previous results are based on the properties of $\widehat{X}_r$ as a consistent and asymptotically normally distributed estimator of x_r under the usual conditions of convergence of Fisher's information (Fahrmeir and Kaufman, 1985).

Furthermore, large sample approximations allow both the construction of confidence intervals and the assessment of different tests for estimating and comparing the parameters of the regression function, the mean or the probability corresponding to the response. In particular, testing the hypothesis H_0: $\beta_2 > 0$ can be of special interest in chronic toxicity experiments since a positive value of β_2 may indicate a non-monotonic trend in the concentration-response relationship. In fact, it is well known that in some situations the test substance may slightly stimulate the viability of a species at very low concentrations before causing toxicity at higher levels (Capizzi *et al.*, 1985).

In conclusion, generalized linear models and particularly binomial, negative binomial and gamma regression models, as suggested in the present paper, appear to offer an attractive approach to the analysis of dichotomous, count and continuous data, respectively. These methods provide an appreciable improvement over the current statistical parametric practices which are still currently used for the analysis of acute and chronic test data. Furthermore, they are easy to handle and allow the use of standard maximum-likelihood methods. However, the main advantage and interest of the methods presented in this work lies in their wide range of applicability which is a consequence of the realism and/or the versatility of the underlying hypotheses and models.

The author is willing to provide listings or a floppy disk containing the programs which enable the calculation of endpoints and confidence intervals by means of the regression methods presented in this paper. These interactive programs are easily adaptable to most experimental designs in acute or chronic toxicity experiments.

REFERENCES

Bard (1974) *Non Linear Parameter Estimation.* Academic Press, New York.

Barndorff-Nielsen O (1978).*Information and Exponential Families in Statistical Theory.* Wiley, New York.

Capizzi T., Oppenheimer L., Mehta H., Naimie H. and Fair J.L. (1985) Statistical considerations in the evaluation of chronic aquatic toxicity studies. *Environ. Sci. Technol. 19*:35-43.

Fahrmeir L. and Kaufman H. (1985) Consistency and asymptotic normality of the maximum likelihood estimator in generalized linear models. *Annals of Statistics 13*:342-368.

Gelber R.D., Lavin P.T., Mehta C.R. and Schoenfeld D.A. (1985) Statistical analysis. In *Fundamentals of Aquatic Toxicology,* ed.Rand G.M. and Petrocelli S.R. Hemisphere, 110-123.

Lawless J.F. (1987) Negative binomial and mixed Poisson regression. *Can. J. Statist. 15*:209-225.

Maul A., El-Shaarawi A.H. and Férard J.F. Application of negative binomial regression models to the analysis of quantal bioassays data. *Environmetrics* (in press).

McCullagh P. and Nelder J.A. (1983) *Generalized Linear Models*. Chapman and Hall, London.

Nelder J.A. and Wedderburn R.W.M. (1972) Generalized linear models. *J. R. Statist. Soc. A*, *135*:370-384.

The Need for Software Validation in Routine Toxicology

H. D. Unkelbach

Fachbereich Mathematik/Naturwissenschaften/Datenverarbeitung
Fachhochschule Wiesbaden
Von-Lade-Straße 1, D-6222 Geisenheim

1. Introduction

The word "need" in the title of this paper "The need for software validation in routine toxicology" is connected with the word "routine". Routine toxicology is considered to be a counterpart of "exploratory" toxicology. Whereas exploratory toxicology looks for unknown toxic effects, it is the task of routine toxicology to exclude toxic effects or to confirm exploratory results. In other words, routine toxicology is understood as that part of toxicology which makes the information on the safety of drugs or the toxicity of chemical substances reliable.

To this aim, toxicologists and pathologists do their best in conducting well-designed and well-planned trials. Biometricians do their best by optimizing experimental design and analyzing the data. One premise for the success of their work is - among others - the usage of reliable and high quality software. To confirm that the software in use is really valid and reliable is the task of software validation.

The quality of information is determined by the quality of the underlying raw data and the procedures processing them. Therefore, as a consequence of the principles of the Good Laboratory Practice (GLP), all software used for a toxicological study is subject to the quality assurance program of the laboratory. It is the user, and not the developer or the vendor of the software, who is responsible for the correctness of the results obtained by the use of the software. Therefore, he must perform systematic and well-documented validation. Specific care must be taken for statistical programs which, in contrast to other software, cannot be validated by simple comparisons of data or simple recalculations by hand, because they evaluate rather complex formulas by rather complicated numerical methods. Because of the large amount of statistical tests in a toxicological study and the decisive consequences of the statistical results, the statistical software used in a toxicological department must be of high quality and extremely reliable. Hence, it must be intensively validated before it is installed for use. One premise for solid validation is that the numerical quality of the software is well-documented. Some requirements on the development process and the documentation of statistical software are discussed.

As the topic of this paper is strongly connected with GLP, a short glance will be thrown in the next section at the actual situation of GLP within the European Community, followed by a rough outline of software validation. Attention is then focussed on the specific aspects of software which is used for statistical evaluation. Commonly used statistical software packages are contemplated with respect to their numeric quality. The shortcomings are discussed and proposals are given as to how numeric quality could be made transparent and, then, be improved.

2. GLP in the European Community

The history of GLP began in 1968/69. The World Health Organization (WHO) formulated the so called "Good Manufacturing Practice" (GMP) principles to give some guidelines for producers of drugs to be considered during the drug manufacturing process (WHO, 1969). Corresponding principles for the research fields, the "Good Laboratory Practice" (GLP) regulations, were declared by the US Food and Drug Administration (FDA) in 1978 (FDA, 1978).

The GLP principles were intended to make the data of safety studies valid and reliable, which gives the basis for reliable information on the safety of drugs. A further aim was to formulate a basis on which the quality of studies could be made clear and studies conducted by different laboratories could be made comparable with respect to their information quality.

It was because of this second goal that the Organization of Economic Cooperation and Development (OECD) adopted these principles. They made it possible for member states of the organization to have confidence in the research of other member states which presented the basis for trade and commerce of drugs within the OECD.

Some years later, in 1987, the Commission of the European Community, too, accepted the principles of GLP which were already in use in many OECD countries (Decision 87/18/EEC of the Commission of the EC, 18. Dec. 1986). In the meantime, further guidelines of the OECD have been adopted by the European Community (88/320/EEC, 89/569/EEC, 90/18/EEC). These include guidelines for:

- monitoring GLP principles,
- inspecting the compliance with the GLP principles,
- conducting laboratory inspections and study audits.

The Commission of the EC also requests the member states

- to establish national procedures for monitoring GLP compliance,
- to designate national authorities to perform the corresponding functions,

- to establish national law.

In Germany, e. g., GLP principles are mandatory by law for Research and Development (R&D) of all chemicals ("Chemikaliengesetz", Neufassung vom 14. März 1990).

The perspectives of the EC to gain a common market with free movement of products go far beyond those of the OECD. Harmonizing the quality standards of R&D work, harmonizing the monitoring procedures for compliance with the GLP principles and harmonizing the inspection procedures is expected to yield

- confidence in the R&D research of other countries

and thereafter

- mutual acceptance of the test results between all member states.

This gives the basis for really free movement of products within the EC and gives equal opportunities of competition within the EC to all producers of drugs. The benefits are not restricted to these points. Consider e. g., that the exchange of reliable information between scientists through all countries and the belief in the quality of research will reduce duplication of trials, reduce the number of animals and, thus, reserve R&D resources for other research.

3. Software validation

Software validation is not explicitly demanded by the GLP guidelines. But it is a consequence of GLP. It is deduced from the guidelines, since any method, procedure or equipment used in the conduct of safety studies is demanded to be validated. This demand covers software as well.

In early times this fact was not realized by many practitioners. At first, the US FDA edited an internal guideline for FDA-inspectors, the so-called "blue book" (FDA, 1983). This internal guideline instructs the inspectors on what kind of validation activities would be required and how computer equipment should be inspected. After some inspections had been performed along the guideline, the existence of the "blue book" became known in the industry. The Quality Assurance Units (QAU) of pharmaceutical companies became aware of the problem of software validation and that this task should be tackled.

This task has been performed since 1983. Although the "blue book" was originally written for the pharmaceutical *manufacturing* field it was also applied to the *R&D* domains. The US Pharmaceutical Manufacturing Association (PMA) as well as the Drug Information Association (DIA) organized large meetings on the new topic of software validation to clarify what must to be done in the industry. This process ended in 1988 after a so-called "Consensus Workshop" had taken place. Scientists, practitioners, people from data processing and FDA worked out a common proposal of what to do. The agreement was formulated in a book (DIA, 1988). The proposals are consistent with the ANSI/IEEE Standards for software validation and also to German Standards (DIN, RAL) (cf. references). Although the "Consensus Book" is not an official guideline of the FDA or any other authority, it can be understood as the broad consensus of competent people on the topic of software validation in the pharmaceutical field.

The main facts can be summarized as follows. *Software validation is an essential part of the quality assurance program of a toxicological department.* The "Consensus Book" (DIA, 1988) gives answers, how this task can be organized and performed.

Up to now, only one reason for the need of software validation has been discussed, namely the official requirements of governmental authorities. But this is a rather shallow reason, and if a more intrinsic reason did not exist, people would indeed believe the regulations to be pure bureaucratism or governmental despotism.

As mentioned in the introduction, the major part of toxicological work consists in routine toxicology. Characteristics of routine toxicology are

- large amounts of data and
- many statistical results.

It is impossible to check each individual calculation and to reflect about each individual statistical test result. The procedures must be performed routinely and also the conclusions must be drawn routinely, one can say, like assembly line work without thinking about the relevance at the time of producing the results. An error causing an incorrect result has no chance to be detected and may have fatal consequences.

Therefore, the procedures themselves must be extremely reliable. Reliability as the main quality characteristic of a system can be made clear by methods of software validation. Hence, *software validation is of primary interest of the user* and not only a requirement of authorities.

In the following, a rough outline of the main topics of software validation will be given. More detailled information can be found in Passing and Unkelbach (1987) and Wolf and Unkelbach (1986).

The definition of software validation is simple and clear:

- **Software validation is giving documented evidence that the software really does what it is supposed to do.**

For many practitioners, the point of responsibility does not seem to be so clear. It is not the developer of a program and it is not the vendor of a software system who are responsible for the application of the software. A scientist who draws conclusions from his study is fully responsible for his result. If the result is wrong because he had used bad software - perhaps, without being aware of it - he is nevertheless responsible. A company has no chance to make a software vendor liable for any disadvantage resulting from the use of the software. Usually, such a warrantee is directly excluded in a normal software contract.

Therefore, *the user himself must take care of all methods and tools* he uses for his work. Governmental authorities, moreover, demand that the user proves that he has taken care. Consequently, *the user has to document* all his corresponding activities.

The objects of software validation are

- the functions,
- the quality characteristics.

The functions of the software must work correctly and reliably. Furthermore, all quality characteristics defined in the specification of the software must hold. The tasks of the user are usually divided into three parts

- the validation concept,
- validation protocols,
- validation reports.

First of all, the user has to formulate and to organize a validation concept for all validation activities he will perform. He has to descibe generally what kind of activities will be performed, at what time points and under what circumstances they will be performed, and how he will performe these activities. This general concept makes up the **validation system** of a toxicological department. It is usually formulated in the form of "Standard Operating Procedures" (SOP's).

Before any actual validation of some functions or some quality characteristics of the software takes place, the user has to define what he is going to do, how he will do it, and what conclusions he will draw from any possible result. He must refer to the corresponding points in the validations SOP's. This gives the **validation protocol** of a concrete validation activity.

After the validation protocol is finished, the validation itself must be performed according to the protocol, and a **report** of the activities and the results including any expected or unexpected event must be written. Also, the conclusions drawn from the results must be documented. Then the user, the in-house quality assurance inspector, or any other inspector from outside would be able to reconstruct or even reproduce what had been done.

Today, scientists in the pharmaceutical industry are generally willing to validate their systems, but have little or no experience. Therefore, people are not exactly certain what they are expected to do. This paper is not intended to give detailed instructions, but if one keeps in mind the aims and main ideas of software validation, one may be able to deduce what must be done in a practical situation.

The main aim of any validation activity is the quality of information. The quality of information is given by

- validity of data,

- safety of data,
- integrity of data,
- reliability of procedures.

First of all, the *data* generated in the laboratories must be valid. Strong precautions must be taken to ensure that data cannot be lost or damaged in any way. The second part of good information is due to reliable *procedures* for processing the data. All steps during the lifecycle of the data must be absolutely safe.

The procedures which are today of primary interest to governmental authorities are the procedures for

- data collection,
- data management,
- transfer of data,
- archiving data,
- documenting data,
- reporting data.

The procedures for

- statistical analysis

seem to be not the primary interest of quality assurance staffs today. (But this may change in the near future.) The reason may be that inspectors today are generally not trained in statistics, and the methods of validating statistical software are rather different from those of other software. The functions of other software can normally be validated by simple comparison of data (data before and after some transformation) or by simple recalculations by hand (sums, averages, products,...). But statistical software cannot be validated by simple methods, because it exhibits rather specific properties.

4. Statistical software

Statistical software is numerical software. It is based on mathematical formulas which are often quite complicated. Formulas usually have restricted ranges of validity. Often several formulas must be used in various ranges which agree in their common margins.

In statistics, approximations and limit distributions are often used instead of exact formulas. But it is often not clear how accurate the approximations are and from which number n the limit distributions can be applied. Furthermore, rank tests are usually valid only for continuous samples, so it remains open how to handle ties.

Another specific feature of numerical software is that figures are represented as floating point figures and that floating point arithmetic is used. Therefore, formulas principally cannot be evaluated to any degree of accuracy. The problem of rounding errors, propagation of errors, loss of digits, or the exponentiation underflow should only be mentioned. Different programming of the same formula can lead to different results. Inept programming can even lead to incorrect results. In particular, iterative methods which converge theoretically may diverge on the computer.

According to the experience of the author, none of the mentioned specific characteristics of statistical software are currently the object of GLP-inspections, and also are not the object of validation. Of course, the developer of statistical programs may have made every effort to solve the programming problems and to work out the complicated formulas in the best way he knows. But, in general, it is not clear to the user or any third party (e. g., GLP-inspectors) to what extent the numerical problems are solved.

This statement is also true for many well-known and widely-used statistical software packages available on the market. They are often of rather limited numerical quality. Many investigations on the reliability of statistical packages have been performed by independent groups. One of these investigations, published by Bernard et al. (1988), compared non-parametric statistical test procedures of some packages. These procedures were found to be unreliable in many cases, e. g., for small sample sizes. Large differences between the different packages were established.

The shortcomings of statistical software packages mentioned above are often more extreme for statistical programs which are supplemented as a marginal component to other non-statistical software. Consider, e. g., data aquisition systems usually installed in toxicological laboratories. Those systems incorporate "report writers" which are supplemented by some statistical programs to mark significant results. Such programs are often developed because of the user's demand, but without statistical or numerical expertise. They are often rather unreliable.

Summarizing these findings, statistical software today is often found to have *no defined numerical quality,* which means that no documentation exists describing the quality characteristics, e. g., the accuracy of results for any possible constellation of data. Therefore, this software is *not ready for solid validation* of numerical quality. The only possibility of getting some feeling of quality consists in testing the procedures by black box testing for some arbitrarily chosen data examples.

At this point, the next problem of testing numerical software appears. What are the correct results of the chosen data examples? The obtained results are often compared with results calculated by corresponding procedures of another alternative statistical package. Or examples are used, for which reference results can be found in the literature. But these testing methods are clearly not sufficient because of the large variety of possible results. Statistical procedures, generally, cannot really be validated by arbitrarily chosen examples.

Instead of black box tests one needs white box tests, theoretical validation or even mathematical proofs of correctness. Consider, e. g., a random number generator. It cannot be tested by simple examples, but by mathematical proofs or, alternatively, by large well-planned, well-organized and well-evaluated simulation studies.

But clearly, such an effort cannot usually be made by the user during his work in practice. Therefore, the problem must be solved in another way.

In the past, numerical mathematicians and statisticians discussed the problems with programmers or computer scientists in scientific terms (e. g., Bernhard et al., 1988). This scientific discussion was not heard by practitioners. They went on buying the well-known statistical packages and accepting the programs as they were. Unkelbach and Passing (1989) suggested that numerical quality should be formulated in terms of software quality assurance like other software rather than in scientific terms. Then numerical quality could also be assured and validated according to software engineering methods like other software characteristics. How this can be done is outlined in the next section.

5. Numeric quality assurance

Software quality begins with the planning of the software. Like any other technical product, "quality is designed in, not tested in" (Taylor, 1985). Therefore the quality characteristics must already be declared at the beginning of the planning process in the software requirements specification.

The **requirements specification** of statistical software should embody in addition to the usual content of any other software

- the basic mathematical formulas,
- the numeric accuracy,
- a priori test cases.

The basic mathematical formulas should be described for any possible data constellation with their validity ranges and with all boundary conditions. The formulas must be explicitly given in algorithmic form as they should be programmed. The numeric accuracy must be predefined for normal and also for all extreme borderline cases. Especially, the number of valid digits must be named. A priori test cases must be chosen carefully such that they will serve as reference values for verfication purposes. If possible, the expected results should be given. At least some simple examples with known results must be available.

If these characteristics are defined during the requirement specification process, it will be ensured automatically that the expertise of statisticians and numerical mathematicians will be involved. Furthermore, the specified numerical properties are the object of care during the developing process, and the requirements which are fulfilled become part of the system description of the software.

The **system description** of statistical software should embody in addition to its content in other software the

- mathematical methods description.

It describes which agorithms are used in any possible data constellation. It contains the reasons why the algorithm solves the problem in question, e. g., with references. Furthermore, the accuracy of any possible result is specified, e. g., by upper and lower limits, and the arguments of all statements must be presented (e. g., references, proofs, simulation studies, plausibility considerations).

If **iterative methods** are used, further information must be given. It must be clarified for which initial values theoretical convergence is guaranteed. Also the numerical convergence must be discussed, e. g., by stability considerations. Finally, the termination criteria of the iterations must be described and established.

The system description is primarily the internal documentation of the software and will not be read by the user during his practical work. He uses the handbook or the manual. Therefore, the manual must contain the main points of numerical quality in order to perform and interpret the numerical results properly.

The **user manual** of statistical software should embody in addition to its content of other software

- the accuracy of results in any range,
- hints, if the reliablity of a result has not been proven in advance,
- test data with the expected results for harmless and numerically hard cases.

There are cases for which the reliability of a result cannot be proven in advance. Consider e. g., iterative methods for some non-linear regression problem, for which it is not known if they will converge or if they will converge to the correct limit value. In such cases, the user must be warned in the manual. Then he will interpret the results carefully. The test data given in the user manual serve for validation purposes by the user, e. g., after the installation.

If all these requirements are fulfilled, the software has a clearly defined numeric quality. The basis is given that the software can be validated in accordance with the actual validation guidelines.

For this purpose the corresponding documentation of the developer

- the methods description,
- the test documentation,
- test data records with correct results

must be available to the validator who may be the user or an academic institute or any official quality institution.

The **proposals** above can be summarized as follows:

- Software validation is mandatory in the toxicological environment.
- The developing process of statistical software should incorporate numerical quality assurance.
- Numerical quality should be clearly declared in the documentation.
- Quality assurance documentation should be available to the user.

If these demands are fulfilled, the software has a defined numerical quality and is ready for solid validation, and not only for black box testing. The benefits will be

- better statistical software,
- more reliable toxicological information, and therefore
- more valid toxicological information.

Remark: The author is aware that the criteria described above are demanding and can only be fulfilled by a considerable effort. A producer of software who is restricted by a limited budget may be obliged to keep his effort low. In this case, however, the gaps in the software quality must be explicitly mentioned in the methods description and the user manual so that the user may interpret the results critically and explain errors, if they occur.

Acknowledgement

The author is grateful to G. Schultz-Herzberger for her help in editing the manuscript and to G. A. Christ, both E. Merck Darmstadt, for valuable hints and discussion on topics of GLP.

References

ANSI/IEEE Standard 830-1983: IEEE Guide to Software Requirements Specification

ANSI/IEEE Standard 730-1981: IEEE Standard to Software Quality Assurance Plans

ANSI/IEEE Standard 829-1983: IEEE Standard for Software Test Documentation

ANSI/IEEE Standard 1012-1986: IEEE Standard for Software Verification and Validation Plans

Bernhard G et al. (1988) Investigations on the reliability of some elementary nonparametric methods in statistical analysis systems. Statistical Software Newsletter **14**: 14-26

Deutsche Gesellschaft für Qualität (DGQ) und Nachrichtentechnische Gesellschaft im VDE (NTG) (1986) Software-Qualitätssicherung, Aufgaben, Möglichkeiten und Lösungen. Beuth Verlag, Berlin

Deutsches Institut für Gütesicherung und Kennzeichnung: RAL-GZ 901 (1985) Software Gütesicherung

DIN Deutsches Institut für Normung e V (1985) DIN 66285 (Vornorm) Anwendungssoftware - Prüfgrundsätze

Drug Information Association (1988) Computerized Data Systems for Nonclinical Safety Assessment - Current Concepts and Quality Assurance. Maple Glen (PA)

Food and Drug Administration (1978) Nonclinical Laboratory Studies, Good Laboratory Practice Regulations. Federal Register **43**, No 247, 59986-60025, 22.12.1978

Food and Drug Administration (1983) Guide to Inspection of Computerized Systems in Drug Processing. Reprint in Pharmac. Industry **1**: 39-68

Food and Drug Administration (1987) A Guide to the Inspection of Software Development Activities (The Software Lifecycle)

Hausen HL (1983) Software Validation. Proceedings of the Symposium of Software Validation. Darmstadt

Meyers G (1978) The Art of Software Testing. Wiley, New York

Passing H, Unkelbach HD (1987) Software-Validierung aus dem Blickwinkel der GLP- bzw. GMP-Richtlinien. Pharm. Ind. **49** : 590-595

Taylor D (1985) Software quality assurance as viewed by quality assurance. Presentation, DIA-Meeting: "Computer Software Validation Techniques", Philadelphia

Unkelbach HD, Passing H (1989) Quality assurance of statistical software. Statistical Software Newsletter **15** : 49-55

Unkelbach HD, Wolf T (1987) RAL-Gütesiegel Software im Gültigkeitsbereich von GLP und GMP. Pharm. Ind. **49** : 916-918

Wolf T, Unkelbach HD (1986) Informationsmanagement in Chemie und Pharma. Teubner Verlag, Stuttgart

World Health Organization (1969) Good Practices in the Manufacture and Quality Control of Drugs. WHO Official Records, No 176, Annex 12, Part 1, 99-104

AN APPLICATION OF MIXED MODEL ANOVA FOR THE ASSESMENT OF MOTOR ACTIVITY IN RAT BEHAVIOURAL TOXICITY STUDIES

P. Repeto , Biometrics, GLAXO S.p.A - Italy

Introduction

The statistical analysis of motor activity in rat behavioural toxicity studies is presented.

The experimental design analyzed was as follows:40 rats were randomly allocated to 4 treatment groups, each group containing 10 rats. Each rat was studied for 20 minutes, with data for a number of motor activity parameters observed through a DIGISCAN and recorded at 5-minute intervals, according to the following scheme:

			TIME (min)			
		Rat no.	5	10	15	20
Treatment	T1	1	Y	Y	Y	Y
		.	.	.	.	.
		10	Y	Y	Y	Y
	T2	1	Y	Y	Y	Y
		.	.	.	.	.
		10	Y	Y	Y	Y
	T3	1	Y	Y	Y	Y
		.	.	.	.	.
		10	Y	Y	Y	Y
	T4	1	Y	Y	Y	Y
		.	.	.	.	.
		10	Y	Y	Y	Y

A very simple way to analyze this experiment would be to perform a one-way Analysis of Variance (ANOVA) , comparing the treatments at each time. This analysis, however, is not able to detect the effect of time and the interaction between time and treatment.

The model proposed in this paper is the MIXED MODEL ANOVA which makes it possible to test: the effect of treatment, the effect of time, and the interaction between time and treatment. The correlation between the observations taken on a rat at different times can thus be taken into account.

Statistical Model

The model employed for this analysis was the following:

$$Y_{ijk} = u + \alpha_i + \beta_j + s_{k(i)} + \gamma_{ij} + \varepsilon_{ijk}$$

where:

α_i = effect of i-th treatment group i=1..4

β_j = effect of j-th time j=1..4

$s_{k(i)}$ = effect of subject k-th in group i ($s \sim N(0,\sigma_s^2)$) k=1..10

γ_{ij} = effect of interaction between i-th treatment and j-th time

ε_{ijk} = error ($\varepsilon \sim N(0,\sigma_\varepsilon^2)$)

α , ß and γ are fixed effects. Each is considered a random effect distributed as $N(0,\sigma_s^2)$, and all are considered independent random variables; ε is distributed as $N(0,\sigma_\varepsilon^2)$. If s is considered a random variable it is possible to take into account the statistical dependence between the observations taken on the same subject (rat) at different times, the correlation coefficient between two observations of the same subject at different times being given by:

$$\rho^2 = \sigma_s^2 / (\sigma_s^2 + \sigma_\varepsilon^2)$$

The above formula shows that the correlation is independent from each pair of time points j_1 and j_2 considered.

The statistical model can also be considered in terms of expected mean square:

SOURCE OF VARIATION	MEAN SQUARE (MS)
TREATMENTS	MS(ERROR) + Q (TREATMENT,TREATMENT*TIME) + Q (SUBJECT(TREATMENT))
TIMES	MS(ERROR) + Q (TIME, TREATMENT*TIME)
SUBJECT(TREATMENT)	MS(ERROR) + Q (SUBJECT(TRATMENTS))
TREATMENT*TIME INTERACTION	MS(ERROR) + Q (TREATMENT*TIME)

Q is a quadratic form depending on the effects involved (in brackets).

As one can see the only estimable effect, when interaction is present, is that of subject (rat) effect, i. e. the variability between subjects. The other main effects, those of time and treatments, are estimable only if the interaction is absent. The strategy of the analysis is to verify whether there is interaction and, in its absence, to test the effect of time and treatment. If interaction is present the only possibility is to compare the treatment at each time.

Examples

As an example the analysis of the parameter "horizontal activity" (number of horizontal movements performed by a rat in a 5-minute interval) will be presented. The table of mean (s.d) values of the parameter is the following:

Tab. 1 Mean values (s.d.) of horizontal movement in each time interval and for each group of treatment

Treatment	Time (min) 5	10	15	20
T1	25.84 (3.75)	19.47 (3.09)	12.49 (3.85)	8.92 (4.54)
T2	22.36 (9.29)	26.15 (4.61)	26.28 (4.65)	26.78 (6.65)
T3	23.12 (6.06)	18.17 (5.83)	17.33 (3.72)	14.49 (4.94)
T4	10.86 (10.45)	6.42 (8.50)	2.98 (4.49)	2.20 (3.81)

The table of the MIXED MODEL ANOVA performed on the data from Table 1 is:

Tab. 2 ANALYSIS OF VARIANCE TABLE

SOURCE OF VARIATION	MEAN SQUARE (MS)
TIME	466.87
TREATMENT	2676.59
SUBJECT(TREATMENT)	80.60
TIME*TREATMENT	154.70
ERROR	19.66

The F test of interaction gives:

F - MS (TREATMENT*TIME)/MS (ERROR)- 7.87 , P-.0001

Fig. 1 gives a graphical interpretation of the significant interaction found in the analysis. It is simple to note that the comparisons between the treatments give different results depending on time.

A case of no interaction effect can be obtained from the first example if we consider only treatments T3 and T4. .

The MIXED MODEL ANOVA decomposition is shown in the following table:

Tab 3. ANALYSIS OF VARIANCE TABLE

SOURCE OF VARIATION	MEAN SQUARE (MS)
TIME	278.02
TREATMENT	3204.85
SUBJECT(TREATMENT)	112.01
TIME*TREATMENT	6.60
ERROR	16.92

The F test for interaction gives F-0.39, P-0.76 n.s. This fact makes it possible to test the overall effect of the difference between treatments using the MS (SUBJECT(TREATMENTS) as the error term. The corresponding F test gives:

HORIZONTAL ACTIVITY
T1
T2
T3
T4
n. of horizontal movements (x 10²)
30
25
20
15
10
5
0
5
10
15
20
Time (min.)

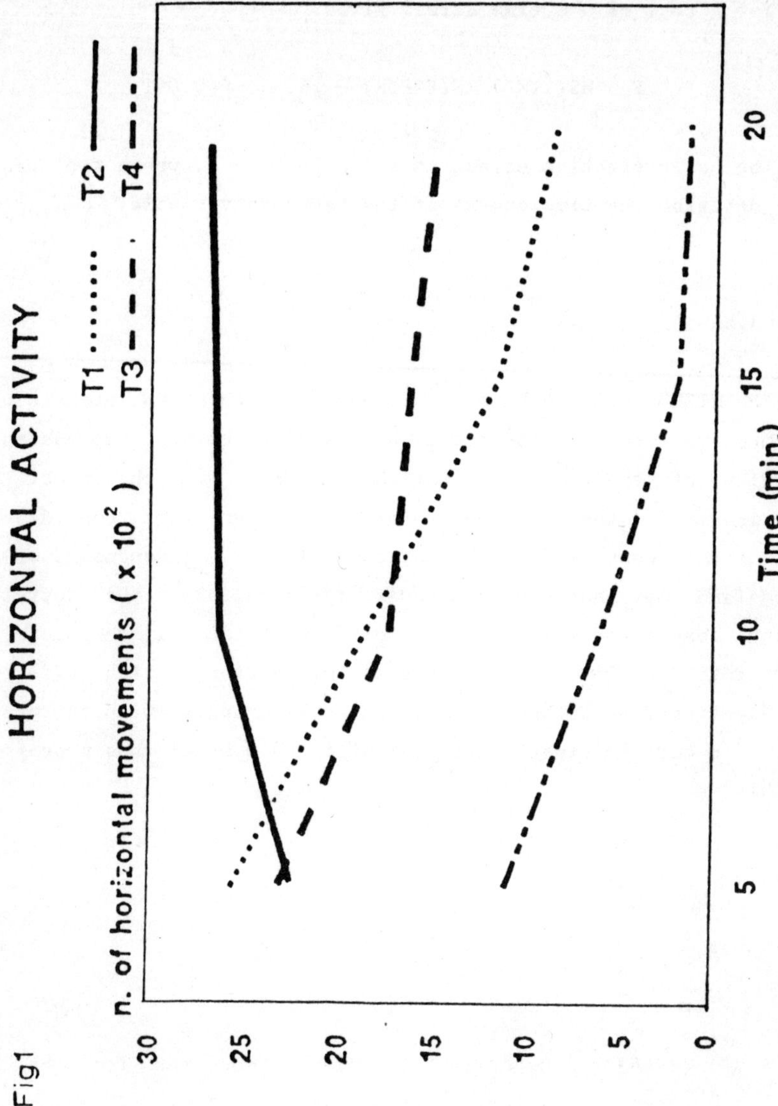

Fig1

The F test of the time effect gives:

F - MS(TIME)/MS(ERROR) - 16.43, P-0.001

The no interaction effect is shown in Fig. 2, where two parallel lines describe the time course of the response variable.

Conclusion

The MIXED MODEL ANOVA makes it possible, when no interaction is present, to compare treatments by means of curves expressing the evolution of the response variable in time. On the other hand, comparisons of the treatments at each given time consider the experimental response obtained at each time independent of each other (and may thus give contradictory results); the correlation between observations performed at different times is, therefore, not taken into account. The absence of interaction, which offers the above-mentioned advantages, can be ascertained only with the proposed model . In certain experimental situation this model thus proves more flexible.

References

Kirk R .E. (1968) Experimental Design: Procedures for the Behavioural Sciences Brooks/cole 171 - 182

Index